400 NAVELS: THE FUTURE OF SCHOOL HEALTH IN AMERICA

By Godfrey E. Cronin and William M. Young

Phi Delta Kappa
Bloomington, Indiana

Photos courtesy of William M. Young & Associates,
Oak Park, Illinois

Cover design by Victoria Voelker

Dedication

This book is dedicated to the courage and optimism of the school board members of the Posen-Robbins Elementary School District 143½ in suburban Cook County, Illinois. These men gave of their time freely, after hours as well as time from their jobs, to bring the school health clinic to fruition in an area where there were little or no school health services. We therefore pay tribute to Henry T. Rogers, president; David Cebulski, secretary; Flenor Clemons, member; Walter Dohl, member; Ronald Jauch, member; Leonard Marsh, Sr., member; Dennis Schnering, member; and Henry Gentile and Leonard Carriere, attorneys for the school district.

Table of Contents

Introduction

by

Adlai E. Stevenson
U.S. Senator, Illinois

It brings me special pleasure to introduce readers to an exciting new concept in school health care delivery that promises to
have important applications both to urban and rural school
systems throughout our country. Although similar ideas have
been tested in several states, I am delighted that Illinois School
District 143½ in Posen-Robbins has had the opportunity to present a unique model that should be examined in terms of public
policy for national health care.

The Office of Child Health Affairs (HEW) states that there
are 250,000 mothers giving birth each year with little or no prenatal care and five to 10 million children today with *no* access
to primary health care.

We must find a solution to help build young, healthy Americans, and schools may well be the cornerstone of that solution.

The innovative model in health care in the Posen-Robbins
schools has been given birth by the Robert Wood Johnson
Foundation, which is committed to the development of a cost-
effective, viable school health care system. At a time when
school budgets are being cut, it is critical to have a permanent
design that involves state-level agencies and private insurers
in financial reimbursement for health care services.

The Posen-Robbins School District 143½ demonstrates that
the marriage of school with health services can be a happy one.
It brings regular health care not only to the poor, but to all
children who go to school. Buildings are in place and clinics
can be set up in unused or remodeled classrooms as the school

v

population declines. Nurse practitioners and paraprofessional health aides are utilized in schools in medically underserved communities to provide a broader range of comprehensive health care and health education to children than previously has been available.

Posen-Robbins is a model that deserves study and further appropriate public and private initiatives. I hope you will find the Posen-Robbins story as significant to the health needs of our children as I have.

Part I: Posen-Robbins

"Perhaps the single most important contribution school health programs can make to promote health is to emphasize the importance of lifestyles and the environment, and to teach each child how to use the health system. Our recent attempts to contain health costs may be successful in the short run. The hope for the future, however, rests with the next generation of health consumers, the children of today."

Joseph Califano
Secretary of Health,
Education, and Welfare

The Bottom of the Bird Cage

If you had to select one symptom that symbolized the inadequacy of health care in the communities of Posen and Robbins, it was the 400 navels.

The 400 navels were discovered back in the mid-sixties during one of the federal government's periodic programs called EPSDT, which stands for Early Periodic Screening and Diagnostic Training. In Illinois we call that program Medicheck, and it's the children's portion of Medicaid, the health care system for poverty families. EPSDT provides physical examinations and some medical treatment under Title I for children from Medicaid families.

Although our school population, like those of other school districts, has shrunk in the decade since the mid-sixties, there were approximately 3,000 students within Posen-Robbins School District 143½ back then. Four hundred of these 3,000 students (13.3%) had umbilical hernias, that is, protrusions of their bellybuttons, some of them up to seven inches long!

Having an umbilical hernia is not life-threatening. It is more a cosmetic than a health problem. It also is more common for blacks to have umbilical hernias than whites. Most umbilical hernias disappear spontaneously, the rest normally are repaired by a pediatrician by the time the child reaches the age of two or three. But as Dr. Eugene Diamond, medical director for the Posen-Robbins School Health Project explains, "The fact that this condition persisted into school age would indicate these hernias were not being repaired at the appropriate time."

It was partly a matter of money. Posen-Robbins is typical of many areas throughout the United States where lack of income makes proper health care—particularly for children—a rarity.

2

According to U.S. government estimates, approximately five to 10 million children in the U.S. are "without public or private sources of comprehensive and continuous health care." The families of these children seek health services and treatment for them only in times of emergency. They also lack access to primary health care that might prevent illnesses. Dr. Charles U. Lowe, special assistant for child health affairs at the Department of Health, Education, and Welfare states: "Of all the dollars in the family, the most elastic is prevention care for children. The health dollar pays for the breadwinner first, the mother second, then the children."

Certain forms of health care that middle- and upper-class families take for granted are unknown by lower-class families. Take, for example, dental care. By the time children reach school age, they have an average of three decayed teeth. One out of three children has gum disease. Approximately half of all children under age 15 never have had dental care.

The key reason for inadequate health care is poverty. Poor children suffer health problems much more than children from families with an adequate income. Children born to families with annual incomes lower than $3,000 are more than four times as likely, according to U.S. government statistics, to have "poor or fair health." They fail to grow as tall. Their blood has a low hemoglobin count. They have a higher incidence of disease. They miss more days of school.

According to HEW's Office of Child Health Affairs: "The mothers of 10% of all newborns receive little or no prenatal care, thereby increasing the risk of subsequent illness and disability to themselves and their infants. Not unexpectedly, the poor persons in rural and inner-city areas and minorities are disproportionately represented in the maternal and infant mortality and morbidity data that reflect insufficiencies of the current health and medical care systems."

So the 400 navels were not symptoms of some dread disease, some fatal malady that would strike suddenly without warning like the Legionnaires disease in Philadelphia. Instead, the 400 navels served as a symptom of a more pervasive problem within the Posen-Robbins community: the lack of adequate health care, which over the decades could be just as devastating in terms of its effect on peoples' lives.

Little was done back in the mid-sixties about the fact that nearly one out of every seven students in Posen-Robbins School District 143½ had an umbilical hernia, because that was simply one problem. Posen and Robbins had many, many problems, most of them directly or indirectly the result of the low economic level of the two neighboring Illinois communities. If you repaired the 400 navels, you could turn your back and a few years later there would be 400 more children with umbilical hernias—or perhaps with other, more pernicious problems.

It took nearly a decade before the school district moved to correct the basic problem symbolized by those 400 navels. This was a unique medical solution, a pilot health program based in school, which in its success might well have a profound impact on the future of school health in America.

Posen and Robbins are unique in themselves. They are two small suburban communities south of Chicago. For many years they were considered the bottom of the bird cage in Illinois. Each year Pierre de Vise, assistant professor of urban sciences at the University of Illinois at Chicago Circle, issues a report listing the socioeconomic ranking of Chicago suburbs in an eight-county area. Out of 201 communities listed in his report released September 28, 1977, in the *Chicago Tribune,* Robbins ranked 201st—and had ranked 201st each year since 1971. Posen ranked 163rd, actually an improvement of its rankings of 193rd in 1975, and 189th in 1970. The median home value in Posen of $20,200 placed that community at a near-bottom ranking of 197th in the housing category. Robbins' median home value was $18,500, which made it next to the last. Out of 1,800 students enrolled in the district during the 1977-78 school year, 1,400 were eligible for and received free lunches under the government-funded program, another indication of the low income level of families with school children.

Posen and Robbins are racially identifiable. Posen (population 5,498) is almost entirely white. Robbins (population 9,641) is as equally black. Both communities lie south of Chicago in an area of urban sprawl, a mixture of industrial plants, shopping centers, vacant lots, power lines, and residential neighborhoods. Posen and Robbins are criss-crossed by expressways. The tri-state expressway cuts across School District 143½ from the east to northwest as it bypasses the city of Chicago. Highway I-57 slices through from the south heading toward Chicago's Loop. In one instance, two schools in the district are only four blocks apart, yet because of expressways, one must drive nearly two miles to get from one to the other.

So fragile are the identities of these two communities that the average individual would drive right through them at 55 mph, having no idea he had done so. He might be aware of Posen and Robbins as being part of suburban Chicago—hav-

4

ing heard one or the other municipality mentioned sometime on the 10 o'clock news—but he would have little idea of their locations, or the thoughts of their residents. Particularly this would be true of a resident of the suburbs of Barrington Hills (west of Chicago) or Kenilworth (north of Chicago) that ranked first and second on the same de Vise survey that ranked Posen and Robbins near or at the bottom. The lives of people in Barrington Hills and Kenilworth rarely touch the lives of those in Posen and Robbins.

Posen is a working-class community, mostly first- and second-generation Polish families, who began settling in the area around the turn of the century. It has small neighborhood stores and taverns, with Saint Stanislaus Roman Catholic Church the center of social activities. The church also sponsors a parochial school that attracts many white children of Catholic families and thus reduces the ratio of whites in the public schools to approximately one in five. Some children from Robbins also attend three parochial schools in nearby Blue Island.

The area was subdivided around the time of Chicago's first world's fair, the Columbian Exposition of 1893. Soon afterwards, Polish immigrant families began settling in the area, getting off the Grand Trunk railroad and dropping their few possessions in the empty fields. They were attracted by jobs nearby at the Ingalls-Shephard factory in Harvey or at North American Car Shop in Blue Island. The Polish people who settled in Posen (named after the city in western Poland, Poznan, from which many of them came) wrote home to their friends and relatives who formed succeeding waves of immigrants.

It was not only the jobs that attracted them, but also the familiarity of the land. For the same reason the Swedes settled in Minnesota, the Poles settled south of Chicago. Walter Dohl, a member of the Posen-Robbins school board, comes from a German background, but after attending a showing of movies and slides by one of the Saint Stanislaus priests who recently made a trip back to Poland, he commented, "The thing that struck me was that so many of the scenes in his pictures were dead ringers for what I remember as a kid around here. You saw a gravel, two-lane street, with a ditch on each side, and a fence made out of little strips of wood, and geese walking down the street. It was exactly the same."

The people settled on the land and built their homes. The freight cars at North American Car Shop were wooden, and when their siding was replaced, the scraps often were carted home on two-wheel wagons to serve as building material. According to Walter Dohl, "You still can go through town and find all kinds of old houses that have stencil marks on them from the railroad cars."

The people of Posen sunk their roots deeply into the land and raised their children, who also settled in Posen and raised their children near the family home. Although people of other ethnic groups gradually moved into Posen, the community retains its basic Polish identity today. The people worked diligently, sometimes in several jobs. Although they did not make much money, they did not often squander it foolishly. As their fortunes improved, they built homes with materials no longer collected from North American Car Shop. The homes in Posen today look comfortable, but they are not sumptuous. The streets are clean. The lawns are well manicured. Aside from the low-level noise of traffic passing on the expressways, Posen is a quiet place in which to live.

The establishment of the adjoining community of Robbins started later. It began during the decades between the two world wars, mostly through the settlement of blacks who migrated to Chicago from the rural south seeking factory jobs, but who did not wish to live under crowded inner-city conditions. George Walker, assistant superintendent for the school district, says, "The people who came here wanted to get back out in the country where they could raise their own food and raise their families in a rural setting, where they thought they had some control. My father wanted to have a home so his children would have a better chance growing up independent."

Robbins was black, born of prejudice, settled by people not permitted to settle anywhere else. Walter Dohl recalls that his father knew several individuals born as slaves. "They didn't have any education," he says. "The land they were sold was not worth much for anything. When I was a kid, you could go up and down the street and there were old quarry holes filled with water and garbage. Robbins had no economic base. The people living there were the last hired and the first fired. The water supply for the entire village of Robbins was a town pump."

Many of the homes were shanties, built a room at a time as their residents accumulated second- and third-hand building materials. The shanties had dirt floors, were heated only by ovens, and were owned by absentee landlords who charged $25 to $35 a month—and even that was too much. Jitney taxicabs provided transportation from the end of the bus line at 139th and Western into Robbins for 10¢ a person. There were no street lights and no sewers. On each side of the streets were open ditches where cars got stuck, yet George Walker looks back on the Robbins of Depression days with a certain degree of nostalgia, "It was a small village of friendly people with one school, the Lincoln school. When something was given at school at night, everyone in town was there. You didn't worry much about locking your doors, because there wasn't much to be taken anyway."

Robbins had fewer than 1,000 people in the thirties, but following World War II the exodus began from the black ghettos on Chicago's west and south sides, swelling the population to nearly 10,000 by 1970. George Walker went away to school at the University of Illinois in 1946, then taught in North Carolina. When he returned, he realized that so many new people had moved into town, he hardly knew anybody now when he rode the bus. The identity of the people was changing, but a single common denominator remained: poverty.

Meanwhile, Posen remained Polish mostly through choice. Robbins remained black less by choice, but because there were fewer neighborhoods into which residents could easily move and be accepted. The migration of the fifties and sixties included not only people on public aid, but also factory workers, post office clerks, and businessmen. Robbins today has three faces: 1) the shacks of yesterday that gradually are being demolished as people move out of them into public housing; 2) inexpensively built private homes in which low- to medium-income families struggle to pay rent or make mortgage payments; and 3) an increasing number of relatively expensive homes in which well-paid professionals live. But this last group is a minority within a minority; most of the people in Robbins are poor.

In the late thirties, with population increasing in the suburbs south of Chicago, the county board decided to divide its former school district 143 in half. Midlothian, a community to the west of Posen and Robbins, more prosperous and with more land for expansion, retained its identity as district 143. Posen was part of an area that was to become the newly designated district 143½, which also encompassed sections of neighboring Markham, Harvey, and Blue Island. Robbins was caught in the middle. Midlothian did not want Robbins because it was poor and black, and neither did Posen. But Posen did want the Libby plant on Western Avenue and a section of railroad tracks in the district because they were taxable property. The county board finally told the people of Posen that if they wanted the advantage of the tax base, they also had to assume the burden

7

of Robbins. Thus was born, from a wedding of convenience, Posen-Robbins School District 143½.

During the next few decades, educational improvements within the newly created district rated low priority partly because of the simple ethnic fact that Polish people are predominately Roman Catholic. Most of their children attended the parochial school sponsored by Saint Stanislaus Church. They had little incentive for improving the public school system. The people of Robbins, still coping with the difficulties of being black in a white society, had not yet made education one of their main priorities.

Because the public school system was ignored, its problems began to multiply. In the early sixties, Posen-Robbins had one of the first teacher strikes in northern Illinois, led by the American Federation of Teachers. The administration fired 21 teachers for not appearing for work during the strike, and when 21 more teachers supported them, they, too, got fired. This eliminated 42 of the 110 teachers in the district. There was tremendous animosity between teachers and the administration at this time, with the teachers often lining up outside the superintendent's office at night with their complaints.

Educationally, the schools suffered from neglect. The district had no regular reading series that served all grades and often had to borrow books from other districts. There were no school libraries. The roofs leaked, windows were broken, and there was an even more critical problem of academic achievement. Standardized tests indicated an average reading level of 5.4 for students leaving high school. Most Posen-Robbins students dropped out of high school by age 16.

The district also had difficulty meeting standards for state and federally supported programs. At one point the state, insisting the district's Title I program did not meet guidelines, threatened to reclaim $150,000 in federal funds. The district eventually settled for a $40,000 repayment with three years to pay. When Posen-Robbins wanted to establish a school lunch program, it learned that in order to qualify for assistance it needed a complete kitchen—at a time it did not even have a hot plate.

"Posen-Robbins had a bad reputation," admits Walter Dohl. "Whenever the local television stations wanted to do a program on how *not* to do things, they came to us. We were bad educationally. The board supposedly was a bunch of crooks. The staff was unqualified. We were just everybody's bad exam-

8

ple. If you wanted to know the wrong way to do something, you looked at Posen-Robbins."

One advantage of being at the bottom is that the only way you can go is up. Posen-Robbins soon was to move upward, a steady ascent that saw it not only improve educationally, but also develop a pilot program for improving the health of its school children that might well become a model for schools all over the U.S.

Genesis of a School Health Program

In September, 1972, the superintendent of schools resigned and, as part of the new administration,* we began to look for some new solutions to the district's continuing problems. Recognizing that Posen-Robbins did not have the economic base to allow major changes from within, we began to look for aid elsewhere. We established a free lunch program, obtained mobile units housing three libraries, instituted a K-8 reading series, and attracted grants to repair neglected buildings. If someone came to us and said you could get a grant to ripen bananas in Posen-Robbins, we would say, "Okay, let's go!"

Posen-Robbins' image soon changed. A career education program begun in the district soon was being distributed to seventh- and eighth-grade classes through the U.S. We also worked more closely with the school at Saint Stanislaus, initiating mutual programs and supplying the parochial school with special teachers, psychological services, and social workers.

Posen-Robbins gradually began to rise from its position at the bottom of the bird cage. Within four years, the average reading scores of graduates from our district increased from 5.4 to 7.2, and the teachers no longer lined up in the hallway outside the superintendent's office with complaints. They were too busy attending classes (paid for by the district) to improve their teaching skills. People soon began to talk about Posen-Robbins School District 143½ as a progressive leader in education.

It was not simply the appointment of a new superintendent that caused this transformation; the district was ripe for change. Much of the credit for implementation of the above

---

*It was at this time that the school board appointed this book's co-author, Godfrey Cronin, one of the district's two assistant superintendents, to be the new superintendent of schools.

programs should go to members of the seven-man school board with whom the administration worked very closely. Posen-Robbins was fortunate in having a board that was totally committed to seeking excellence in education. The main contribution of the administration was to get a diverse group of people involved, pull them together, and make things happen.

One key element in the upgrading of the school system was the involvement of more and more parents. At one stage two mothers came to see us, frustrated at what they considered the general lack of health in the school children. They had been examining the health records of children in the district because of a new law passed in Illinois in the early seventies requiring every student entering school, as well as those entering fifth grade, to have a physical examination on file. The majority of the students in our district had no physical examinations on file, and those that were on file were frequently incomplete. We had only 28 days to fulfill the state requirements, otherwise we would have to begin excluding children from school.

Fortunately, with the use of funds from the Title I ESEA program, we were able to hire a resident doctor at one of the Chicago medical schools to provide the physicals in time. We paid $5 per physical examination, which of necessity had to be limited in scope. But what the doctor discovered while giving those physical examinations was what disturbed the mothers. She discovered children who were partially sighted, hard of hearing, and with various other maladies. In a few instances, children assigned to special education classes were not mentally retarded, but rather were deaf.

Merely identifying these health problems, or in the case of several children, reidentifying the problems that had been discovered during the earlier program when the 400 navels were noted, did little toward solving them. The problems were simply listed in the medical records of the Posen-Robbins school children, but nothing happened. The mothers felt there should be more follow-up.

This was less a fault of the Medicheck program as it applied to Posen-Robbins—or as it was applied in the state of Illinois—than it was a symptom of neglected health screening programs nationally. Legislation to set up the Early Periodic Screening Diagnosis and Treatment Program was passed by Congress in 1967 to try to prod state and local health organizations to pay systematic attention to the health needs of poor children who suffer from anemia, deafness, eye defects, and a host of other health problems at a higher rate than would be expected from the general population. Although the EPSDT program served children and youth to age 21, it particularly was geared to those under six.

The EPSDT program had lofty goals when established in 1967 and its designers anticipated that 13 million underprivileged children might be served by it. Alas, by July, 1974, seven years later, only 1.5 million had been given medical examinations. According to figures from Dr. M. Keith Weikel of the Bureau of Medical Services, Social and Rehabilitation Service, a division of the Social Security Administration, almost none received any follow-up treatment. The following year the federal government announced penalties totaling $1.7 million (reductions in their welfare aid) for seven states that failed to implement the EPSDT programs.

Posen and Robbins, because of their low economic base, were the type of communities toward which the Medicheck program had been directed. "There never has been any sort of continuing care in the school district," explains Dr. Eugene Diamond. "Through use of Title I funds, we were able to transport some of the neediest children to hospitals for treatment of the problems we identified, but after that was done, we sat down and asked ourselves, What are we going to do next year? How can we bring decent health care into the community?"

"There are no doctors in Robbins," explains Dr. Diamond. "There have been a few sporadic start-ups in the form of medical care, episodic things such as clinics that would convene a few times a week. A doctor committed to another community would spend some time there, but none of these efforts succeeded, at least not during my 20 years in the area. Posen has had limited care in that time. It now has a small group practice with one or two individuals, but the school district taken as a unit never has been adequately cared for by resident physicians."

What the people of Posen and Robbins often did was to seek health care only in crisis situations. They utilized the emergency room at St. Francis Hospital in Blue Island, a larger community to the north. This was an inefficient and expensive means of obtaining treatment. Dr. Diamond suspects that at least 50% of visits to the St. Francis emergency room could have been handled by a doctor at his office, *if* the patient had some kind of continuing relationship with a local physician.

"Our emergency room partly serves as a clinic for people who don't have private physicians," he says. Some people obtain treatment at public clinics at Cook County Hospital west of Chicago's Loop, often sharing the 24-mile taxicab ride with other ill people. Dr. Diamond calls this "the 10 dollar illness," because you have to be sick enough to be willing to spend 10 dollars for the taxicab ride downtown.

Such health care not only is more expensive than it would be if there were a neighborhood health center available, but it often is less effective. "There is no follow-up," says Dr. Diamond, "so usually you get noncompliance when you recommend therapy. The result is a recurrence of acute problems or perpetuation of chronic problems, because nobody is counseling the patient or seeing to it that he follows through on instructions. Not only that, they are charged twice as much in an emergency room, because of the extra staffing needed, than if I were delivering the same kind of care in my office." But the people of Posen and Robbins had no other choice—until the school system became interested in providing them with health care.

In upgrading educational facilities and programs at Posen-Robbins, we had been working with a number of consultants and source people.* One of the programs involved students from Chicago State University working with teachers in the classroom, called Cooperative Urban Teacher Education, but better known as the "CUTE" program.

During a meeting related to this program one afternoon, we discussed the lack of Medicheck follow-up and the concern of the mothers. The result of our discussion was a decision to try to come up with some program to upgrade the health of students in the district. We speculated that if you could improve the health of students, you also might be able to improve their academic level, since they would be absent less often and be more able to concentrate on their lessons while in school.

This discussion brought us back to the previously asked question: how can we bring decent health care into the community? Could the school system be involved? The basic problem that people most think about is money. Decent health care costs money. The cost of proper medical treatment in the U.S. is very expensive and growing more expensive each day.

But more money is available than many people realize, even within the school system. There are at least a dozen federal agencies (according to a report prepared in November, 1976, by the Office of Child Health Affairs) providing earmarked funds totaling more than $2.1 billion to state and local agencies for

---

*One of them was this book's co-author, William M. Young, formerly dean of education at Chicago State University, now an educational consultant with offices in Oak Park, Illinois.

13

school health activities. And there are general health funds that may be spent for the same purpose. The mechanism at least is available at the federal level for funding health activities. Unfortunately, there is little coordination and joint planning among the above agencies.

In addition to the above-mentioned $2.1 billion, there is an estimated $300 million that the states provide for school health activities, although again with little coordination or priority. Thirty-five states administer school health services through their state education departments, but 11 of these states have no one person responsible for health services. Fifteen states and the District of Columbia have school health programs administered by a combination of state agencies.

So money is available, and health care can be obtained when needed. But this poses no guarantee that such health care *will* be obtained. As the Office of Child Health Affairs points out in one position paper: "The experience of England and other countries indicates that even removal of the need for payment at point of service does not in itself bring into the system the poor who may need care the most."

Improving access to this system for that group seemed to us an exciting challenge. We thought we could utilize the facilities of our school system to improve public health. Of all the institutions in the country with roots in the community, the school system is the most accessible and can be most responsive to community needs. Politically, it is one place where the man on the street can have some direct input. The school system is not so far removed from the people that they can't have an effect on its policies. This was particularly true in School District 143½ where the seven members of the school board were average men who had been elected by their neighbors.

The school board at this time included: Henry Rogers, the president, black, a community action specialist serving four states for the Department of Health, Education, and Welfare; David Cebulski, the secretary, white, an independent businessman; Flenor Clemons, black, an independent businessman; Walter Dohl, white, an engineer for the Gulf and Western Railroad; Ronald Jauch, white, an independent businessman; Leonard Marsh, black, an employee of Argonne National Laboratories; and Dennis Schnering, white, an independent businessman. They provided a good cross sampling of the communities of Posen and Robbins, and their support would be essential in the months of planning to come.

In March, 1974, we met with Frank Jones of the Robert Wood

14

Johnson Foundation. We questioned him about the possibility of trying to deliver health care in what might be considered a nontraditional system. We considered the political and economic barriers that would need to be overcome. Jones felt that we would need the complete support of the school board and administrative staff. One important question was, Who would pay for it? While schools constitute a channel through which health care delivery is possible, very few public schools offer health services other than those provided by school nurses. But most school nurses are so limited by both school regulations and tradition that they cannot dispense even aspirin without a parent's approval, so their usual response is not to diagnose, or treat, but simply to send home. Starting an in-school program would pose a gamble in light of the above problems, but if Posen-Robbins could demonstrate that it worked, it would open up possibilities for health care delivery in many other nontraditional medical care centers.

Later, we met with Dr. John Hall, director of the Cook County department of public health. After discussing several ideas with him related to improved health care, we decided to see if we could get support from one of the charitable foundations for a project in this area.

We wrote letters to the three area hospitals and asked their administrators to meet with us and Dr. Hall. Administrators of two of the hospitals came to hear us formulate a plan to provide health care through the school system, possibly in cooperation with the hospitals and possibly with the involvement of medical students. The two administrators did not seem eager to shoulder this burden. They left us with the idea that their personnel already were overworked and we were getting in over our heads.

In June, 1974, we submitted a document to the Robert Wood Johnson Foundation suggesting an experiment in providing health care in the Posen-Robbins school district utilizing two groups. One group would receive health care within the school and another control group would receive no health care other than what they normally received through parental initiative. We anticipated using the children in a purely experimental situation to assess their health status and to determine whether improving their health level would increase their educational level.

By August we met again with Frank Jones. The Robert Wood Johnson Foundation strongly opposed using control groups in such a situation because it meant some children would receive care and others would not, creating an unequal situation. Out of this meeting came the decision to drop the idea of a controlled experiment and instead to establish a comprehensive school health delivery system that would benefit the entire district.

For the next six months we worked on a proposal that would establish and fund health care for youngsters in Posen-Robbins. The more we worked on the proposal, the more apparent it became that we needed more time to plan such a program. This led us to request funds from the Robert Wood Johnson Foundation to support a planning grant.

In March, 1975, the foundation sent a team of site visitors to Posen-Robbins to determine whether the district should be awarded the grant. Included in that first team were: Phil Nader, from the University of Texas Medical School in Galveston; Bert Fischer, a sociologist from the University of Wisconsin; Frank Jones from the Robert Wood Johnson Foundation; and Christine Grant, another program officer from the foundation.

We decided at that meeting that because the children of the district were not getting primary care in the community, the school system could deliver that care. The group did not think at this time that the plan would become a model for other districts. They saw it almost as serving a charitable need because the school district was so poverty-stricken.

During this time we received the full support of the school board. On three separate instances, board members got up for a 5:00 a.m. meeting at O'Hare International Airport with people from the foundation, then went to their own jobs, then came back at 1:00 p.m. for further discussions. The Robert Wood Johnson Foundation eventually approved the planning grant and in July, 1975, the Posen-Robbins school board committed itself to support the program. The planning grant would run for one year from August 1, 1975, to August 1, 1976.

We decided that the first thing we wanted to do in planning the project was to see what other people were doing around the country. We needed information on school nurses, school doctors, and an exciting new breed of health care providers who went by the name of school nurse practitioners. We also learned of three projects that involved delivery of health care at the school level in Cambridge, Massachusetts; Hartford, Connecticut; and Galveston, Texas. In September, accompanied by Dr. Hall and school board member Walter Dohl, we visited the first two cities, and we visited the third soon after.

It was the beginning of active research into the future of school health in America.

Part II: Health Professionals View School Health

Nurses and the School System

"One of the most wasted resource persons in the health care field today is the school nurse," declares Judith Igoe, project director for the School Nurse Practitioner Program of the School of Nursing, University of Colorado. When we decided to examine how health care could be delivered in a school setting, she was one of the key people we talked to. She added, "School nurses are underutilized, sometimes undertrained, yet potentially they could provide health care for millions of school children and, in so doing, help raise their capabilities for learning."

Igoe's views, we learned, are shared by many school health professionals and health organizations across the nation. According to the American Nurses' Association, there are now 30,000 school nurses in the U.S. employed directly by school districts. In addition, several thousand public health nurses devote part of their time to school health. With 91,000 public schools in the country this means there is one nurse for approximately every three schools, however, there is a maldistribution of nursing personnel. According to Stephen J. Jerrick, executive director of the American School Health Association, affluent school districts may have more nurses than they need, while poverty-area schools and also many middle-class area school systems frequently have neither nurses nor any semblance of a school health program.

As we traveled the nation exploring the world of school health, we discovered that the caliber of school nurses varied from state to state and from one school district to another. Some states require that a school nurse have a bachelor's degree and advanced training in community health. Other states require only that a school nurse be a registered nurse; and in some states there are no certification requirements whatsoever. Such variations, of course, reflect the many-faceted educational patterns of the nursing profession, which include three-year diploma schools as well as college degree programs.

Many school districts perform only those health services required by law, while others have gone ahead with innovative programs such as those involving the school nurse practitioner, who through advanced training is competent to perform some of the traditional functions of a physician.

In addition to the poor distribution of school nurses, there also is a shortage of school physicians. Fewer than 500 full-time doctors specialize in school health in the U.S., and many of them spend most of their time on administrative tasks. Meanwhile, according to Igoe, the average school nurse spends only about 25% of his or her time in the actual delivery of health care to children. Anywhere from 45 to 65% of a school nurse's time is devoted to clerical chores.

The school nurse shortage is not one of manpower. Jerrick believes there are an adequate number of nurses, although they may not yet be trained in adequate numbers to fulfill the new roles to be discussed later in this book. Nevertheless, the reluctance of many school boards to allocate funds for hiring them and to implement school health programs constitutes a widespread problem that may be solved only if and when Congress enacts a nationally coordinated child health plan, including school health.

Even when a school district initiates a school nurse program, nurses often are burdened with an inordinately large number of children to care for. Organizations such as the American School Health Association and the Department of School Nurses of the National Education Association recommend a nurse-student ratio of one-to-750 or one-to-1,000. Yet even some of the best school health programs fail to approach this ratio. For example, Chicago public school nurses, all with four-year college degrees and advanced training, work with a student-nurse ratio of 3,000 to one. In other school systems, one nurse may have to cover three or four schools, with traveling time reducing effectiveness.

Restrictions placed on the nurse by state or local laws represent perhaps the most fundamental problem in school nursing, we discovered. Despite recent progress in upgrading the status of school nurses, they all too often remain dispensers of Band-Aids and keepers of records. One nurse who formerly worked in a school system in a small town in Texas told us, "The health program in that system was simply pieced together, and the people in education had a different idea of what a nurse should do than I did. They felt a nurse was somebody to be available quickly if someone bleeds."

William B. Schaffrath, director of the National Joint Practice Commission, an organization concerned with developing better collaborative efforts between nurses and physicians, observes, "State laws, and restrictions often imposed by local medical societies and school boards, severely limit what the nurse may do in the schools. Legally, the nurse usually may only 'assess and manage,' which means she can't diagnose and treat. If she does, she could be charged with illegally practicing medicine." Lorrine Glazebrook, a school nurse at Valley High School in Des Moines, Iowa, and the NEA Department of School Nurses delegate to the American Medical Association's Medicine/Education Committee on School and College Health, adds, "Schools often are afraid that parents may file liability suits, so they tie the nurses' hands. In Iowa, for example, it's even illegal to give a student aspirin or vitamins without written orders from a physician."

However, Judith Igoe offers a much more liberated view of what a competent school nurse could do to provide better health care for students. She states, "If the school nurse is to provide care with competence and efficiency, he or she must be able to: develop a health history, perform general physical and psychosocial examinations, make primary diagnoses and assessments, evaluate environmental factors and community resources, and initiate and modify regimens of care."

The question of how much responsibility a nurse should have is a matter of controversy in school systems and among health officials. In some schools, the trend in the last decade has been to relieve the school nurse of routine duties and to view that person more as a pivotal member of a school health team. Some of the more forward-thinking school systems (but still too few) train teachers to handle minor first aid and to use school aides for clerical duties. This frees the school nurse not only to handle common childhood illnesses and emergencies but also to devote more time to the implementation of screening and immunization programs, health education, and student and parent counseling. The school nurse whose talents are properly utilized can be the catalyst who brings together many diverse people and groups. Jerrick says, "We have always considered the school nurse to be the most important individual in the school health program. She is the coordinator among the school physicians, school dentists, school psychologists, school counselors, speech pathologists, teachers, parents, boards of health, voluntary health agencies, medical communities, family physicians, and the health education program in the school."

The ideal, unfortunately, seldom is the reality. According to the American School Health Association, only 23 states have mandatory nursing certification requirements requiring a four-year college degree and advanced training in community health. The most progressive programs can be found in New York, Illinois, Washington, Colorado, Pennsylvania, and New Jersey, with many of the least advanced programs in the south and southwest. Ten states have "permissive" requirements that vary but fall far short of the mandatory standards, and 14 states have no certification standards for school nursing.

Despite problems, the school nurse's role slowly has improved in recent years. School nursing goes back to 1891, when a physician attending the International Congress of Hygiene proposed that a staff of specially educated nurses should visit England's schools to examine children. In 1897, California became the first state to place nurses on a municipal payroll, employing them to visit schools in the Los Angeles area. At about the same time, two public health nurses in New York demonstrated how the assignments of a school nurse could affect the absentee rate due to student illness. The program proved so successful that the New York City Health Department organized a municipally sponsored school nursing service. In 1920, New York State passed the first law requiring nurses to take college courses in education, a move that many other states eventually adopted.

In these early years, school nurses primarily were concerned with preventing the spread of communicable disease, applying minor first aid, and handling medical emergencies. In many schools, this role has continued unchanged for some 80 years. Anyone over 40 remembers the lady in the white uniform with the thermometer and tongue depressor, urging every student to say "a-a-aaah."

By the end of World War II, there were 7,000 school nurses in the U.S., but in the next two decades, that number tripled. In 1965 Congress passed Title I of the Elementary and Secondary Education Act, which provided federal funds for expanded school health and other related services. Within one year after passage of that law, 5,000 new school nurse positions were filled. With federal funds available, many retired registered nurses returned to work while others left hospitals for school jobs. Even isolated rural schools employed nurses for the first time.

This rush into school nursing also created problems. Hospital-oriented nurses, accustomed to their traditional white garb and patient care roles, found that most schools wanted them to dress like teachers and direct health care was often secondary to other duties. They suddenly realized that their three-year nursing diplomas were insufficient for school work. Where required by law, many began to take college courses in education, community health, and related fields. Nevertheless, according to the American Nurses Association, only one-third of school nurses today fulfill the four-year degree standard.

Different preparation is not the only factor that distinguishes the ideal school nurse from her hospital counterpart. Personality also must be considered. "Hospital nurses function under close supervision," explains Dr. Donald E. Cook of the American Academy of Pediatrics. "Community health nurses, including those in schools, are more comfortable in a less-structured environment and like to work independently. They are more attuned to the need for prevention rather than caring for the sick. And, of course, they must like children."

Many school nurses hired after passage of the Elementary and Secondary Education Act later discovered that the federal funds were really "seed money" to enable schools to *begin* health programs to be financed later out of local funds. When the federal money ran out, some schools dismissed school nurses. The failure in recent years of school budget elections has resulted in further cutbacks in, or sometimes complete elimination of, school health services.

Still, in the past 10 years, the number of school nurses has grown by some 10,000. One reason is the new Education for All Handicapped Children Act, which provides federal funds for development of school programs, including school nursing services, for mentally retarded and other handicapped children. Much of the growth in the total number of nurses has been in those states requiring four-year degrees, especially among affluent school districts providing extensive school health services. Many private schools also have hired nurses in the past decade for the first time. But in the inner cities, and in cities of all sizes where school taxes cannot generate enough revenue, the school health picture and the status of school nurses is a sorry one.

"Seven million of the more than 55 million school-age children in the United States never have visited a doctor's office, clinic, or hospital except in cases of extreme illness or emergency," says Igoe. "Millions more have emotional disturbances, perceptual handicaps, speech problems, and similar difficulties. Good professional care is available, yet these children never have gone to a place where such care is administered."

In many states, the only school health care mandated by law is immunization and screening for hearing and vision defects. Sometimes not even that is required. In Arizona, for example, hearing screening is required but not vision screening. Some schools with limited or nonexistent health programs rely on public health nurses to do just enough to meet the state's legal requirements. Even when a screening program does exist, it often contains no provisions for remedial care, a particularly acute problem in low-income areas.

How important is screening? A study by the American Academy of Pediatrics indicates that 5% of all first-graders have vision defects and recommends that screening should be performed each year throughout elementary and high school years. Similarly, the same percentage of children fail their initial hearing tests. The AAP recommends that hearing testing be performed each year in the early school grades, biennially in the upper elementary grades and at least once in junior and senior high schools. Since many state laws have no such requirements, a number of schools have minimal testing programs. In the better school health programs, nurses or technicians supervised by nurses usually do the screening.

At least 25 states require that some kind of physical examination be performed either by a school or private physician when children enter school and periodically thereafter. Most states require both a general physical and special eye examination; about one-fourth require hearing or dental examinations. The results of proper screening examinations often uncover an unusually high percentage of children with defects. For example, a screening of 30,529 children in San Antonio, Texas, uncovered 2,780 children with abnormal vision. Out of 9,390 screened with an audiometer for hearing defects, 291 had abnormal findings. In Kirksville, Missouri, medical students at the Kirksville College of Osteopathic Medicine screened 30,000 school children each year. "We find that 5% to 10% of the children have a potentially referrable problem," notes Dr. James R. Stookey, dean of the college.

Chicago has developed one of the best school nurse programs in the nation. Besides the legal requirement of a four-year degree, Chicago teacher-nurses (as they commonly are called) also must have 18 semester hours in education and at least nine hours in community health nursing. In addition, more than half of the teacher-nurses have master's degrees in nursing education or guidance and counseling. The Chicago school system employs 180 school nurses to serve approximately 525,000 students, but despite the high ratio of 3,000 students to each nurse, and the fact that most nurses must cover two to seven schools, the Chicago program works well largely because it uses trained technicians for vision and hearing screening and school health aides, most of them students, for clerical work.

Jeri Rose, one of the nursing coordinators for Chicago's schools, states, "We have been successful mainly because our technicians and school health aides free our teacher-nurses to perform other tasks, such as follow-up on medical referrals, counseling, and health education." She adds that one of the nurses' major activities is to assist classroom teachers in early identification and referral of children with health problems and procedures for emergency care. This is done through in-service meetings with faculty.

Half of Chicago's students are black and another 15% come from Hispanic backgrounds. As part of an overall integration program in Chicago public schools, the nursing staff includes a proportionate number of black teacher-nurses but still lacks sufficient staff of Hispanic background. To compensate for this shortage, many teacher-nurses take Spanish courses on their own time. Furthermore, many school aides speak Spanish, which helps reduce the language barrier.

Unlike the law in many states that prohibits school nurses from administering medication, Illinois law allows nurses to do so in school as long as they have written permission from the family physician and parents. Thus, Chicago's teacher-nurses have a role in direct health care as well as in preventive health by giving students immunizations against such diseases as diphtheria, polio, tetanus, whooping cough, measles, and rubella. They also assist teachers in setting up health education programs, serve as liaison with parent and community groups, counsel students, and work with both teachers and other school staff in referring children with health problems to proper sources of care.

Another outstanding school nurse program is in the Seattle public schools. It has been in operation since 1908, and presently is headed by Dr. Vivian K. Harlin, a past president of the American School Health Association. Fifty nurses care for the city's 65,000 students, a workable ratio of about 1,300 to one. Besides giving inoculations for numerous diseases and conducting hearing and vision screening programs, the Seattle nurses also check for orthopedic defects and skin diseases, treat allergies, and deal with emotional problems. As in Chicago, they also dispense medication to students under the authorization of a physician.

"Seventy-five percent of all our students either have family physicians or go to a health clinic," says Harlin. "If they have no source of care, we check with the family to assess their income and obtain qualified care for the child on a pay-what-you-can basis. Our nurses also work closely with school health educators by previewing films and books, offering advice, and serving as resource people. In addition, they counsel teachers and help students with health problems that may range from obesity to drug abuse."

As in Chicago, Seattle nurses are on the same salary schedule as teachers. Most are long-term employees, and there are many more applicants for school nurse positions than there are job openings. Besides training teachers, the Seattle nurses constantly seek to improve their own skills through inservice programs conducted by outside medical experts.

Seattle, like other progressive school systems, has begun to utilize school nurse practitioners, a new breed of specially trained nurses. All 50 nurses in the general program have four-year degrees, but three also have school nurse practitioner training and are used for special tasks, such as in-depth assessments, special education programs, and advanced health care that previously would have been performed only by school doctors.

The Chicago and Seattle school nurse programs are strong partly because state laws make it mandatory that the schools use only bachelor's degree nurses with backgrounds in community health. However, some school systems in the states with weak laws have fashioned outstanding programs in the absence of mandatory legislation. In Texas, for example, no school health services except immunization are required. Yet such cities as Houston, Dallas, San Antonio and, most notably, Galveston, all have excellent programs.

The Houston Independent School District serves 210,000 children, 40% black and 20% Mexican-American. There are 140 school nurses, a ratio of about 1,500 to 1, which Houston school officials hope to reduce eventually to 1,200 to 1. The racial ratio among school nurses approximates that in the student population, in compliance with a court integration order. In Houston, every high school and junior high school utilizes one full-time nurse. At the elementary level, no nurse is assigned to more than two schools. Although Texas law requires only that a school nurse be a registered nurse, Houston demands a four-year degree and also requires that its school nurses meet each week for an hour-and-a-half of inservice training.

"Our program operates under a system of objectives," says Virginia Thompson, director of school health services. "We set up specific goals each year and usually meet them. For example, we attempt by the end of each school year to correct 70% of all the health problems detected in screening, and we hope eventually to correct all of them. Our other objectives are to have 80% of all students clearly show an improvement in their health knowledge and to have 95% compliance by the date we are required to report immunization results to the state."

Despite the fact that Texas law requires no school physical examinations, Houston sends as many students as possible to physicians' offices. Nurses do the exams on the remainder of the students. Subsequent referrals for treatment result in the success ratio stated above. In addition to the 140 regular school nurses, Houston uses seven school nurse practitioners in special education of the handicapped and in a children's outpatient clinic funded by the city and county. Among their duties are taking comprehensive pediatric histories.

The situation in Arizona resembles that of Texas in that state laws on school health are almost nonexistent. There are no certification requirements for school nurses, no law requiring physical examination for school entrance, no requirements for health education at either the elementary or secondary levels, no laws mandating that a school hire a nurse, and not even a law requiring vision screening in the schools. Furthermore, Arizona is the only state that has not implemented a Medicaid program, which in some states offers the only health care available for children from poor families. Yet despite these obstacles, the Bureau of Maternal and Child Health of the Arizona Department of Health Services has helped to develop a statewide school health program that brings services into even the most remote villages.

Georgia Macdonough, school health consultant for the Bureau of Maternal and Child Health, has worked throughout Arizona to implement health programs in as many schools as possible. "We're doing the best we can without the help of state law," Macdonough observes. "We don't have enough four-year degree nurses, but we have 900 nurses working in schools. Some schools have full-time registered nurses on staff, but usually an R.N. must serve several schools. We do use public health nurses extensively as well as licensed practical nurses who work on Navajo reservations and are able to speak the Indian language. Some of our nurses are volunteers whose children attend the school where they work. We even have eight nurses who, strictly on their own, have received the training needed to become licensed school nurse practitioners." Despite problems, Arizona has managed to keep its student-nurse ratio near 1,500 to one.

Health service programs differ at the college level as do the duties of the nursing staff. Since colleges must take the place of parents, college nurses have many more duties than do nurses in the public schools. About half of all U.S. colleges have fewer than 1,000 students enrolled, yet even the smallest ones usually have well-developed health services.

There are approximately 3,300 senior and junior colleges in the country, with more than 400 of the larger ones being members of the American College Health Association. V. Arthur Stevens, that organization's assistant executive director, says that almost every college has at least one nurse and the part-time services of a physician. The growing trend among larger colleges is to hire nurse practitioners who can perform many of the duties that a student would expect from a family physician. They often work with a staff of four-year degree and registered nurses, but it is the nurse practitioner who has most of the responsibilities.

If the colleges and some of the more progressive elementary and secondary schools are any indication, it is indeed the school nurse practitioner who may represent the future wave in American school health services. Meanwhile, the position of the school doctor is presently undergoing great change.

How Doctors View School Health

At the beginning of the 1976-77 school year, the New York City Department of Health slashed the budget of its Bureau of School Health by $1 million. It was the latest in a series of budget cuts that, over the years, had forced the city's schools to reduce drastically their health personnel.

Twenty years ago, there were approximately 350 physicians and 800 nurses working in the New York City schools. With this most recent budget cut, Dr. Olive Pitkin, director of the Bureau of School Health, had to terminate 85 physicians, some of whom had been working up to 20 hours a week in the schools. She replaced them with school nurse practitioners. At this writing, there are now only 67 part-time school doctors in New York City, but the number of school nurse practitioners has increased to 78 out of a total nurse force of 200.

The dismissed school doctors were angry; many of those remaining were skeptical about the ability of nurses to replace physicians; and the city's medical community watched the experiment with interest. Today, says Pitkin, school doctors have accepted the nurse practitioners and there has been no negative reaction from outside medical people.

But some of the doctors who lost their jobs remain bitter. Dr. Adele Engelberg, who had worked for 17 years in the city's poverty areas, stated in an article in *Medical Economics,* "They're replacing doctors with nurses, and these women simply are not qualified to do what a doctor does. They can't diagnose cases, they don't know how to take a medical history, yet they walk around with instruments trying to play physician. Many of them even refuse to work without a nurse's aide's assistance, where I often worked alone. New York is setting a very dangerous precedent."

The school nurse practitioner and the school physician are both controversial figures on the educational scene today. As budgets are cut, schools have been forced to trim the cost of their health services, and one method has been to hire nurse practitioners. In New York City the nurse practitioners are all public health nurses with at least two years experience and a year of special training at Cornell University-New York Hospital School of Nursing as nurse practitioners (or pediatric nurse-associates, as they are called in New York).

While school physicians in New York City received $21 an hour for their half-day sessions, nurses now earn about half that. They do routine physical examinations, take histories, provide immunizations, and screen children with suspected problems. Engelberg claims that she frequently had to do physical exams in seven or eight minutes, but that the nurse practitioners usually take half an hour. Pitkin, however, explains that examining nurses always have physician consultation available, and children needing diagnostic work or treatment are referred to family physicians or city health agencies.

As we spoke with medical people across the U.S., we became aware of a strong undercurrent of resentment against any change in what had been considered the traditional role of the school doctor. Although the American Academy of Pediatrics has no formal statement opposing the use of school nurse practitioners, some of the Academy's more influential members question not only their value but also that of the school physician. Dr. Robert Burnett, chairman of the AAP committee on manpower, declares: "We did a survey of our members, and they overwhelmingly rejected the idea of using nurse practitioners in the schools. They may have some value as health educators, but the problem is that they want to hang stethoscopes around their necks and deliver medical care. I feel the same way about school physicians. They might be acceptable as administrators, but they can't do much else. By law they usually can't dispense medications, and all they really do is provide episodic care. For example, what happens to a kid who gets sick at night? Where's the school doctor? Schools have enough trouble teaching, let alone setting up medical care systems."

Another key AAP member, Donald E. Cook, chairman of its committee on school health, agrees: "I think there's a place for nurse practitioners in schools, but cities like New York make a big mistake when they use them on a massive basis. They can function only under a physician's supervision, never independently. Basically, I don't think they're getting enough training. Even in a nine-month college program, such important areas as guidance and counseling often are overlooked. As far as school physicians go, I think that probably any school district with 50,000 or more students needs a full-time medical director to plan and coordinate a health program. The problem comes when a school decides that it's going to give direct medical care."

William H. Carlyon, director of the Department of Health Education of the American Medical Association, observes, "Schools are not proper settings in which to practice medicine. That should be done in a hospital, clinic, or doctor's office where you have the proper staff and equipment. Children should be treated by their family physician or, if they don't have one, at a clinic or through Medicaid. The schools can fill a health role by having nurses, teachers, or technicians provide screening for vision and hearing. There's a place for the nurse practitioner and the physician in such areas as administration and handling of medical emergencies, but the important thing is that a system of health care continuity for the child be developed outside the school. The school's principal concern should be that the child be healthy enough to learn to be a good thinker."

Dr. A. Frederick North, professor of pediatrics and public health at the University of Pittsburgh, is another critic of most traditional school health programs. "The best health role that a school can play is to serve as a matchmaker, getting the child to the right place for treatment," he says. "However, I think that this can be done just as well by public health people as by school personnel. I'm not against nurse practitioners. In fact, I think they usually can do more than a school physician, but I feel that well-trained public health personnel and lay technicians can do a better job than either the nurse or the doctor. School districts, I believe, should use outside medical consultants instead of staff health people. I don't think they need full-time physicians and nurses, and I think they'd be better off if they stayed out of the health business entirely."

Such criticism is regarded by most school health professionals as being outmoded and old-fashioned. Schools would be less likely to enter the health business if it were being run properly. Yet a vast number of medical people around the country apparently react negatively to any suggestions that adequate health care can be dispensed outside the traditional doctor's office.

William B. Schaffrath, executive director of the National

Joint Practice Commission, offers this analysis of the enemies of school health programs: "Many of the opponents of school health systems, particularly pediatricians, are afraid they will suffer financial losses because of competition and also feel their status will be threatened. They don't like school doctors because they think they'll take their business away, and they simply don't understand what school nurse practitioners can do. The fact is that school physicians usually are prohibited by law from offering direct treatment. About 95% of what most school doctors do is really nursing, and this is where the nurse practitioner can be of great value. Working together as part of a team that includes teachers, screening personnel, and others in the school, they can uncover health defects in children and refer them to outside physicians for care. A good school health program means more business, not less, for the outside doctor."

Stephen Jerrick contrasts the role of the private physician with the school doctor largely in terms of preventive health as opposed to direct treatment. "A school health program can succeed only if it has community support," Jerrick told us. "It's not sufficient to rely on the family doctor, because many families don't have private physicians. When outside medical people, whose primary concern is direct medical care, oppose school health programs, they really are opposing preventive medicine. And as far as nurse practitioners go, many doctors just don't realize that practitioners' advanced training relieves the school physician of many routine chores and enables him or her to do a better job of building a school health program centered around prevention."

The history of the American school physician actually is one based on preventive medicine. In the late 1800s, such major cities as New York, Philadelphia, and Boston sought to control such diseases as diphtheria and tuberculosis by hiring doctors to detect suspected victims of these scourges. By the early 1900s, their efforts had proved so successful that communicable diseases affected only 2% of school children. Some schools relied on public health physicians, while others hired their own doctors. Soon the schools began to turn to more comprehensive medical inspections and health services aimed at noncontagious conditions affecting eyes, ears, nose, throat, teeth, and chest. By the 1920s, 26 states had laws related to school medical inspections or health services, a development hastened by the discovery of so many physical defects among young men inducted into military service during World War I.

School physicians continued their involvement in detecting

illnesses through the 1930s; their numbers declined only when school nurses and teachers took over many screening tasks during World War II. Recent studies give estimates of approximately 500 full-time school doctors in the U.S., but even this estimate may be too high. Jerrick estimates that about half the so-called school doctors in America work primarily as administrators. In at least one-third of the nation's 16,500 school districts, according to a study by the U.S. Public Health Service, public health personnel instead of doctors serve the schools. The remaining school districts utilize nurses or outside physicians as consultants. As a general rule, only the larger school districts employ full-time doctors.

The Bureau of Labor Statistics estimates that the U.S. needs about 22,000 new physicians a year, but American medical schools currently graduate only about 15,000. Some observers cite the apparent shortage of physicians as a principal factor for the shortage of school doctors. However, Dr. Burnett, a member of the American Academy of Pediatrics manpower committee, which studied the problem, comments, "There's no shortage of doctors in this country. There may even be too many of them. But there is maldistribution. The affluent communities have sufficient physicians, but there's a real problem in the inner cities and many of the rural areas." Cook, who heads the AAP school health committee, sees an adequate number of physicians available for school work but points to low salaries and school budget cuts as the primary reason for the relatively small number of full-time school doctors.

According to a 1977 survey in *Money* magazine, the typical income for established physicians is $58,000, far ahead of veterinarians, who are in second place at $35,000. Jerrick estimates that the medical director of a large city school system usually starts at $25,000 to $30,000 and seldom goes much above $35,000, except in a major city like Chicago where the medical director earns $45,000.

However, money apparently is not what attracts most physicians into school jobs. Many are pediatricians or family practitioners who desire a less hectic work schedule as they grow older. Others are younger doctors seeking something other than a clinical practice. The school hours and liberal vacations appeal to some. Schaffrath of the National Joint Practice Commission says, "It takes a special type of physician to go into school health work. There are some who don't like surgery and actually can't stand the sight of blood. Others like to be around children or prefer administrative work. I think the vast majority, though, are men and women who prefer preventive medicine to clinical, one-on-one practice, although there are some school doctors who do both. For many, it's more satisfying to make certain that 10,000 children are healthy than to care for only one child at a time."

The American College Health Association estimates that only 200 of the nation's 3,300 senior and junior colleges have full-time medical directors, although most of the rest have part-time arrangements with private physicians. V. Arthur Stevens, assistant executive director of the association, observes: "Traditionally, colleges hired older doctors who were about to retire and wanted to slow down. More and more, however, younger physicians are going into colleges right out of medical school for about one-third what they could make in private practice simply because they like the hours and the intellectual stimulation of the campus."

But even for those doctors willing to make less money to work in schools, frequently no job openings exist. Jerrick anticipates a trend toward using nonphysicians to serve as administrators of school health programs. Philadelphia, which has one of the largest school health services in the nation, already has taken this step.

Under state law, Philadelphia must oversee the health of 359,000 children in 430 public, private, and parochial schools. Before 1960, state funds paid for the entire school health service, but now local school taxes must fund 80% of the cost. Consequently, massive cuts have occurred in the school budget: $8 million in the 1975-76 school year, another $6.5 million cut the following year. As a result, the school system dismissed 10 nurses, four dentists, three clinical physicians, a number of clerical people, and abolished the post of medical director. The former director, Dr. Jerold M. Aronson, left the schools to join a health maintenance organization in Philadelphia, his post being filled by Samuel Kravitz, a nonphysician with 16 years of experience as a Philadelphia school administrator.

"I had been administrator of health services since 1970, so now I'm really filling two jobs," Kravitz explains. "I have access to medical consultants, so I don't feel handicapped by not being a physician." Even with the budget slash, Philadelphia still retains a large number of health personnel. Besides 307 full-time nurses, there are 34 doctors (half M.D.s, the other half osteopaths) who work a minimum of 15 hours a week in the schools, and some hold full-time positions elsewhere. "If we had the money, we could hire all the doctors we want, especially pediatricians," says Kravitz. "With the declining birth rate, many physicians find their business is declining and they'd like to get into the school system, but we just can't take them." Indeed, as we learned from discussions with many individuals, the declining birth rate and its apparent threat to the security (and incomes) of physicians may be a major reason for the opposition in some medical ranks toward school health programs that rely on nurses instead of doctors.

Philadelphia uses its school doctors primarily to perform comprehensive physical examinations in the schools. Previously, these were done in grades one, six, and eleven, but budget cuts resulted in elimination of the eleventh-grade examinations. The Philadelphia school doctors do not provide direct treatment. When they uncover health defects, they refer the child to the family physician, a clinic, or a Medicaid program, as is the custom in most school systems. The doctors also perform skin tuberculin tests, handle medical emergencies, and provide consultation both to parents and school authorities. The school nurses screen for vision, hearing, and growth at least six times during the child's school career. Ten dentists and 14 dental hygienists perform dental screening in grades one, two, and five, and run a dental health education program for children in kindergarten through grade six. When needed, the schools may also call on a corps of 40 psychologists employed by the city's Division of Special Education.

"We have 34 doctors and we really need 52 for the kind of job we'd like to do," Kravitz notes. "Nevertheless, even though we employ so many physicians, we have no conflict with the medical community because we do not perform either direct medical or dental care. In fact, we are probably the biggest provider of patients for private physicians. Besides the cases we refer to outside medical sources, we send all our school athletes to outside doctors for examinations."

Philadelphia may have good relations with local physicians for yet another reason. It is one of the few large school systems that has not yet begun to employ nurse practitioners, thus avoiding an area of potential controversy. Philadelphia stands in sharp contrast to the Chicago Public Schools in this respect.

In addition to employing 10 nurse practitioners from accredited university programs, the Chicago schools also employ an additional 17 trained under special courses devised by medical director Dr. Irving Abrams. They are used primarily in programs financed through the Elementary and Secondary Education Act and other federal funding sources. "I was the first school medical director to use nurse practitioners," claims Abrams. "That was back in 1967, long before the universities even had thought of the idea."

When we were considering what kind of health professionals to employ in our small school district south of Chicago, Abrams told us he felt nurse practitioners receiving extensive nine-month training in formal college programs did not have sufficient instruction to work in the schools. He was convinced of the superiority of his own "pediatric nurse-associates" who, over a 22-week period, receive two-and-a-half hours of weekly training from pediatricians in a local program under which they receive academic credit from the National College of Education in suburban Evanston.

Unlike the medical directors of other big city school systems such as New York and Philadelphia, Abrams has used physicians sparingly in the Chicago schools with only 12 employed on a full-time basis. Four work for the Board of Education to perform pre-employment teacher and civil service health examinations; only eight actually work in the schools. Chicago has four district diagnostic centers, all in inner-city areas, which accept referrals of students with health problems uncovered by the city's teacher-nurses. Each center is staffed by two physicians (a pediatrician and a psychiatrist) along with other members of a health team that includes a teacher-nurse, social worker, psychologist, and nurse practitioner. Two of the nurse practitioners have formal university instruction, while the other two trained in Abrams' program do not. The students receive thorough medical examinations, then are referred elsewhere for treatment.

In addition to the eight school doctors, the Chicago system employs a full-time optometrist, Dr. Mario Rubinelli, who supervises the vision screening program. The schools also retain, on a half-day-a-week basis, the services of an ophthalmologist, otologist, neurologist, allergist, and cardiologist. Their principal function is to examine the records of children with apparent health problems discovered in the schools and to offer consultation to the teacher-nurses.

Despite some controversy surrounding Abrams (not everyone in Chicago health circles believes in the capabilities of his nurse practitioners), he has started some programs, notably in the area of screening, that could be used as models by other school systems. For example, Chicago schools employ 34 full-time, trained testers for vision screening and an equal number for hearing. This deployment of personnel frees the teacher-nurses

35

to perform more significant tasks. Rubinelli says that they test 295,000 students (more than half the total school population) for vision each year. With such intensive screening, they identify vision defects in 20% of the children, a ratio about twice that uncovered in most school screening programs.

When they uncover a defect in a child, the parents receive a call to come in for a conference, at which time they are given a form to take to an eye doctor or clinic. Thanks largely to follow-up by the teacher-nurses, 85% of the children identified as having defects are treated in the first year and most of the remainder the next year. Although Illinois law requires vision screening in only the first, fifth, and ninth grades, Chicago has added another test one year after the first exam. With double testing in the early grades, they catch most defects before the child advances to the third grade.

In a similar fashion, the hearing program, supervised on a part-time basis by Dr. Louis T. Tenta, an otologist in private practice, tests 300,000 children a year at the levels of preschool and grades one, three, five, and eight. At least 20,000 children fail the hearing test each year, again a high enough ratio to suggest that many school screening programs that are less thorough reach only a fraction of the number of children who need medical help.

Naturally, we were most interested in learning how such a program could be duplicated elsewhere. Most observers informed us that optimum benefits from a school health program can be achieved only when there is full cooperation among the medical director, the school health employees, the local medical community, and parents. One physician who has built such a program is Dr. Jerome Newton, director of school health services for the San Antonio Independent School District.

Newton, a pediatrician, worked in private practice in San Antonio for 23 years and also served in the Peace Corps before taking the job of school health director in 1972. The program serves 64,000 children in 90 elementary, junior, and senior high schools and is staffed by 49 school nurses, a dental hygienist, three full-time psychologists, three psychologist associates, three reading specialists, three educational diagnostic specialists, three speech pathologists, three nurse practitioners. A cadre of outside medical personnel work part-time in the schools, including a dentist and eight physicians whose tasks include athletic examinations, supervisory work, and physical examinations in three pupil appraisal centers for children with learning disabilities.

Newton has introduced several innovative programs including one in an often neglected area, dental care. San Antonio stations a mobile van for one full week at each school to conduct dental examinations. Through such concentrated examinations, the dental personnel discovered that half of all the children in kindergarten through grade five require dental work. In addition, under a new program started in January, 1978, through a contract with the public health department, the schools are taking a health census of all preschool children in San Antonio. Half are being examined by school and public health personnel, the remainder by private physicians or in clinics. Through this effort, Newton believes every preschool child soon will have had a thorough examination before entry into kindergarten.

The schools also are launching a program for children with long-term health problems, such as epilepsy or diabetes. The nurse practitioners will act as liaison between school, physician, and clinics for 200 children from lower income families enrolled in the program. "One of the big problems in school health is to find a 'medical home' for children from poor families who don't have private physicians," Newton explains. "A lot of what we do is to obtain continuous care for these children." On his own, he also conducts a clinic on learning disabilities at Santa Rosa Hospital. By offering so much of his time in addition to his formal duties as school health doctor, Newton has built a solid relationship with local private physicians.

One of the best examples of community involvement in a school health program is in Tacoma, Washington. With only 30,000 children in the school system, Dr. Roger Meyer, administrative director of the division of health for the public schools, heads up a program in a city that normally would be regarded as too small to hire a full-time school medical director. Yet Tacoma has had a formal school health program since 1916, and the board of education has always supported it financially. Between 1966 and 1976, a decade when many schools were cutting back on health services, the Tacoma annual school health budget soared from $190,000 to $900,000.

Meyer supervises 80 full-time employees, half of them health educators (an extraordinary number for a school system of any size), and the other half school nurses. Thus Tacoma has a student-nurse ratio of 750 to one, far superior to that recommended by most national health organizations. Five of the nurses have received nurse practitioner training. Meyer believes in the concept. "I think the nurse practitioner is a person whose time has arrived, and the nation's schools must commit themselves to their use."

Like other school physicians, Meyer believes that every child should be treated by his family doctor when possible. Yet in Tacoma, he estimates, one-third of all families with children of school age have no regular source of medical care. As a consequence, Meyer has built a close working relationship with the local medical society and with private physicians. He uses a dozen "team doctors," volunteer physicians who each spend four hours a week in the schools. Their role is purely diagnostic, primarily with children referred by school nurses. Treatment is performed outside the schools. Community facilities, such as the YMCA, are used for children who need special physical therapy. Besides the staff nurses and volunteer physicians, the Tacoma schools also retain the part-time services of a dentist and an ophthalmologist who prescribes glasses for children referred by the vision screening program.

Meyer, whose own background is in public health and behavioral medicine, regards the critics of school health services as years behind the times. "Some physicians say that school health care should be left to private medicine and public health personnel," he states. "However, schools usually are the best available resource for mass screening, immunizations, and referrals to physicians. From my own background, I believe that public health personnel offer only marginal services. A public health doctor generally will go into a school only if there is an epidemic. Public health nurses don't understand school work and don't have the daily contact with children that school nurses and teachers do."

Meyer visualizes an improved school health program built largely around an expanded use of nurse practitioners. They would do more work in poor neighborhoods, assist in crippled children's clinics, offer emergency medical treatment when a doctor is not available, and perform an increasingly important role in mental health counseling. "Many surveys indicate that between 20 and 30% of all school children have emotional problems severe enough to seriously affect their school work," Meyer points out. "The trained nurse practitioner, who deals with the child every day, can be of major assistance not only in the field of mental health but in many other areas. Nurse practitioners should be in charge in many cases, but it's the doctors who have the clout and the laws often state that a nurse practitioner may function only under the direct supervision of a physician."

The future of the school doctor appears to be a question mark.

The number of physicians working in schools continues to decline. An example is Los Angeles where Claude Dapremont, medical director for the Los Angeles Unified School District told us: "We've had to tailor down our services. Like most cities we have been hit by lowered budgets, which results in diminished access to physician services. Physicians who could make more money elsewhere began leaving us. We have dropped from 100 physicians to about 40. We don't do as much as we used to."

Dr. Charles U. Lowe, special assistant for child health affairs at HEW, feels that doctors must change. He says, "If they don't shape up and start figuring out a different role for themselves, an expanded role, they are going to disappear from the school market." But he adds, "There's definitely a need for pediatricians in the school systems as specialists and consultants—which is what they are trained to do."

Lowe recognizes the opposition in certain medical circles and believes that where doctors are opposed to the expanded use of school nurses, it is because of two basic reasons: 1) loss of income, and 2) loss of control over the quality of health care. He notes that in the areas where school health programs have begun to function best, it usually is in a vacuum of medical care caused by the absence of sufficient physicians. "Whether these programs can prosper in areas where there are lots of physicians, we don't yet know," he admits.

Nevertheless, doctors in school systems are increasingly rare, and as schools continue to tighten their health budgets there will be fewer openings for school doctors in years to come. Some schools will rely on nurse practitioners to replace them. Others will turn to nonmedical personnel for administrative work. Some will abolish school health programs altogether. Perhaps it also is time that the school systems of America begin to examine the qualifications of the doctors they hire to run their programs. The era of the old-timer retiring into school work appears to be passé, but is the advent of the young school doctor with no clinical experience any better?

Whatever the direction of school health, there is a growing consensus that medical schools must begin to add school health training to their curricula. "I don't know of a single college faculty pediatrician who has a school background," says Chicago's Dr. Abrams. "Any pediatrician, or any other physician, who plans to work in school health should be required to take a six-month residency in a school before he's allowed to become a school doctor."

The Tacoma school system already has begun such a program, and if it works it may serve as an example for the medical profession. Each year, Dr. Meyer and his health personnel offer school health training to approximately 50 medical students and resident physicians as part of their formal medical instruction. This program is being offered, at no cost to the Tacoma taxpayers, largely because of Meyer's conviction that the job of school physician is becoming so sophisticated that special residency training is mandatory.

But even if trained specialists begin to supervise school health programs, the crucial question remains: once it is determined that a child has a health problem, where do you get medical care? In communities where families have their own physicians, or where there are adequate community clinics, the problem is not a serious one. The real difficulty comes in inner-city and other poverty pockets, as well as in rural areas, where there are limited medical facilities and where parents lack the resources, education, or motivation to get their children the needed care.

The health problems of the poor supposedly were solved when Congress passed the Early Periodic Screening, Detection, and Treatment (EPSDT) portion of Medicaid, which was intended to provide continuous health care for all children of welfare parents. Funded at $137 million in 1977, President Carter recommended an increase to $345 million in 1978, under an expanded program to be called Comprehensive Health Assessments and Primary Care for Children (CHAP).

Dr. A. Frederick North, of the University of Pittsburgh, wrote the EPSDT guidelines, and he remains one of the most outspoken critics of the complex law. "The legislation is written so that federal funds will match state aid, but the administration of the law is left up to each state, and the implementation of Medicaid varies all over the country."

North expands on this subject: "Congress passed the law, many states did little or nothing, and in 1972 Congress declared that the states had to provide health screening for school children from welfare families or pay a penalty. Most of the states conformed. They did the screening, but there was no follow-up. The trouble with EPSDT is that while it provides for a bunch of health examinations, there's no real effort to get a child into continuous care."

The failure of EPSDT, North believes, is its link to Medicaid. To be eligible, a child must have parents on welfare. But as family providers drift in and out of employment, their eligibility for Medicaid assistance fluctuates. And with this change in status, a welfare family may find its children eligible for Medicaid care one week and ineligible the next.

"Medicaid health care is reaching only about 20% of the children who need help," North asserts. "The CHAP expansion of the law might provide for more treatment, but I just don't think the whole thing is going to work. A national health insurance program would help all health programs, including those in the schools. But in the long run, there's going to be the same problem. Physicians simply cannot afford to accept a large number of Medicaid patients, and this leaves the schools and the poor families to depend on nonprofit clinics and a few good-hearted doctors. There's got to be a better way."

Administration, diagnosis, and health education—these are the traditional functions of the school physician. But treatment, no! Either it is not allowed by law or it is avoided for fear of alienating the local medical society and its members. School doctors can do their organizational best, hire scores of nurses or technicians to do screening, perform immunizations, and set up elaborate school health education programs. But in the final analysis, the question comes down to the effective delivery of health care. For at least one of every four school children, the answer is clear. The schools, private physicians, and Congress can't—or won't—do the job.

For one solution to the problem, perhaps those guiding the direction of school health in this country should travel, as we did, to Denver, Colorado, to talk with Dr. Henry K. Silver, a professor of pediatrics at the University of Colorado, and an individual who has had, and will have, a profound effect on the delivery of health services in America primarily because of his espousal of the use of nurse practitioners. Silver has written: "Although it would be of value to have school health care provided by school doctors, there are less than 500 full-time doctors specializing in school health in the U.S. and they, of necessity, must spend a significant portion of their time and effort on administrative responsibilities. In contrast, there are approximately 29,000 school nurses in school health programs who, instead of providing health care and services, presently spend a considerable portion of their time on assigned clerical and administrative tasks."

Silver believes that if we could only tap the true potential of these school nurses, we could make major improvements in the delivery of health care to children in this country. How this idea can, and is, being pursued will be explored in the following chapter.

Extending the Role of the Nurse

Nurse practitioner: those were key words, as we learned while examining the health needs of America. Most of the new, significant school health programs we have seen are built on the shoulders of one or more nurse practitioners. In fact, the utilization of nurse practitioners has emerged as one of the most intriguing health innovations during the last decade in America.

This new breed of health professional working in hospitals, clinics, private practices, and now in schools, has helped to both free the overworked physician from routine work and to provide better and more personalized care for patients.

Depending on the area, a nurse practitioner may go under a slightly different title. To cite a few of the designations we encountered, nurse practitioners sometimes are known as nurse clinicians, nurse associates, pediatric nurse associates, nurse specialists, extended role nurses, certified nurse midwives, or, more commonly in our field, school nurse practitioners. The media sometimes refer to them as "supernurses." Basically almost all varieties of nurse practitioners are registered nurses who are qualified to perform some of the tasks previously considered the perogative of physicians, specifically the diagnosis and treatment of minor illnesses.

In some places, they may even wear the white coats usually associated with "doctors." Other nurse practitioners wear light blue coats, which supposedly identify them as being slightly different from the white-frocked doctors with whom they work. Still other nurse practitioners function in ordinary street clothing. But they all fill different roles than they did as registered nurses.

Sometimes patients have a difficult time telling the difference between the nurse practitioners and the doctors with whom they work in joint practice. And it is not merely the color of the coat each wears. Patients usually associate the use of instruments—stethoscopes for listening to the heart or otoscopes for examining ears—with doctors. Today, nurse practitioners also use these instruments and do other things that nurses previously were not allowed to do.

In some instances, nurses simply are getting recognition for things they have been doing for years. In talking with one nurse practitioner during a visit to Galveston, Texas, we asked if the old-time school nurse was out of date? "No," was her quick reply, "because when you go through a pediatric nurse practitioner program, you just improve your skills. We were doing many of these things as a school nurse before, but we simply have sharpened our skills, which makes us better school nurses. A nurse practitioner maybe can do a better health assessment or evaluation, but I wouldn't say that all school nurses are going out of date."

Nevertheless, they have taken on greater importance in the delivery of health care to people for whom it was unavailable before—within limits. One thing that most nurse practitioners cannot do, because of legal restrictions, is to write prescriptions. Most state laws prevent anyone except a licensed physician from writing on a prescription blank.* That is law, but in practice many nurse practitioners prescribe medication even if not legally permitted to do so. They do this in several ways. After examining a patient and deciding what medication to recommend, they sometimes will ask the physician they work with to write out the prescription. Since most joint practices are built on mutual trust, the physician usually concurs. In some cases, that physician may have signed a number of prescription blanks and entrusted them to his nurse practitioner. Not everyone connected with nursing considers this a good idea.

While in many hospitals throughout the U.S. nurse practitioners visit patients or "make rounds" in the same sense that doctors do, other hospitals prevent them from doing so. Or, if the nurse practitioner does make a patient visit, he or she may be prohibited from writing on the charts to record the patient's progress—even though floor nurses write on those same charts. But as physicians and hospital boards become more exposed to the work done by nurse practitioners and see their capabilities for delivering excellent care at a certain predefined level, old restrictions are lifted. Also, doctors who have employed a nurse

*Idaho and New York recently have modified their laws in this respect.

43

practitioner in their private practice, or who have become involved in working with one in a hospital or clinic setting, find themselves willing to entrust the nurse practitioner with increasing responsibility in the area of patient care.

Some physicians have been slow to accept nurse practitioners because they are so involved in the demands imposed on their own time, that they have not stopped to think about what tasks the nurses could perform if given not merely extra training and proper guidance but an organizational structure in which to work. One Michigan physician we spoke with admitted he only had a vague idea of what nurses did other than give shots, pass pills, and hand out bed pans, until his own wife entered nurse's training. He said that in medical school most doctors have no contact with nursing students, and only rarely do they make rounds together as residents. There is very little joint practice. "Though people claim the nurse and doctor are a team," this physician insisted, "the truth is they often don't even know what the other is thinking."

One worry expressed by people both inside and outside the medical profession is that care obtained from nurse practitioners may be "inferior" care. After all, the typical medical doctor in America has had four years of college, four years of medical school, and anywhere from three to five years as an intern and resident, plus specialty training before hanging up his shingle. Although much research has been done, there is little definition yet as to how much additional training a registered nurse must have before being accepted as a nurse practitioner. Many nurses obtain their R.N. with only three years of study beyond high school, and some nurse practitioners obtain their positions without necessarily obtaining extra schooling. They gain their new skills through on-the-job training.

Admittedly, classroom education cannot substitute for practical experience, but until recently there has been no generally accepted standard for what qualifies a person as a nurse practitioner. The first programs at major universities preparing R.N.s as nurse practitioners were about four months long. Recent certificate programs last nine months, and graduate programs run from one-and-a-half to two years. Regardless of training, the crux of the matter is the amount of confidence each individual physician has in the nurse practitioner with whom he or she is in joint practice. And eventually, it comes down to the confidence the patient has in that physician and nurse practitioner working together. So far, judging from the experience of the pioneers in the field, the physician/nurse practitioner team seems to be working in most instances.

Certain individuals, not entirely familiar with the roles being played by nurse practitioners in health care today, still think of them as "physician's assistants." This includes many practicing doctors, not all of whom have been convinced that they can, or should, upgrade the skills of nurses. A casebook published recently by the National Joint Practice Commission, seeking to promote the acceptance of nurse practitioners by physicians, subtly tried to suggest that doctors who worked with them could improve the care of their patients and could benefit in two other significant areas: 1) they could increase their net profit, and 2) they could delegate many routine medical procedures which they don't find attractive anyway. No doubt nurse practitioners would find these arguments for expanding their skills much less compelling.

The original concept of the nurse practitioners and various other health paraprofessionals emerged at a time when health policy experts worried that there would be too few physicians to care for America's future health needs. The intent of spawning nurse practitioners and other health paraprofessionals, however, was not to create different levels of medical care, but rather to organize a system that identified different tasks to be done and that recognized that these tasks did not necessarily have to be performed by a physician.

Doctors traditionally had "allowed" nurses to take temperatures, weigh patients, and record what they discovered. Many physicians believed that training a nurse practitioner merely meant expanding the number of tasks that a nurse could competently perform, as well as showing the nurse how to perform more complicated tasks. But many nurses object to being thought of as merely physician's assistants who function in some sort of secondary or inferior role. "The role of the nurse is to make the system work for the patient," states Carmela Cavero, a member of the California Joint Practice Commission, "and that's why I object to being called a physician extender, or a physician's assistant. I don't think we are that. I think we're the patient's assistant."

The nurse practitioner movement began in the early 1960s when Dr. Henry K. Silver, a professor of pediatrics at the University of Colorado School of Medicine, became concerned about what he felt was a significant shortage of health care for children in the U.S. Because one of the reasons was the lack of physicians—or more often, their maldistribution in areas where they were most needed—he began to look toward the nursing profession for a solution. He decided that if the role of nurses could be expanded to include some of the basic tasks that occupy physicians' time, more and *better* health care could be provided for all Americans.

"I formulated a plan," recalls Silver. "You started with very skillful registered nurses and give them educational experience in the care of children, so they could have an expanded role and provide care. It seemed to me a very simple idea."

In fact, the idea seemed so simple that Silver at first assumed someone must have tried it before. He spoke to several faculty members at the adjoining School of Nursing at the University of Colorado. They told him they would check and see what they could learn. Silver noticed that the senior nurses with whom he spoke seemed unenthusiastic about his idea and when, after some time passed, they uncovered no information about expanded nursing programs, he began making his own inquiries. He did find several sections of the country in which other individuals had proposed similar expanded roles for nurses. One was in Vermont, but the idea was abandoned because of lack of proper personnel. In Miami, a similar idea had withered for lack of funds. "It became apparent," says Silver, "that nothing had happened, nor would it happen unless individuals from both the nursing and medical profession became interested enough to work together."

In early 1965 Silver had a meeting in his office with Loretta Ford of the School of Nursing at the University of Colorado. He told Ford his concept for expanding the role of nurses in patient care. "Nobody seems interested in it," Silver told her. "Not that they're against it; they're simply not very supportive."

Coincidentally, Ford had been thinking along similar lines. The previous year she had attended a conference where several nurses had discussed the possibility of expanding the role of nurses in offering treatment. Within a few mintues Silver and Ford agreed to begin a program to develop what later would become known as nurse practitioners.

Ford was in charge of public health nursing at the school and supervised a number of graduate nursing students with baccalaureate degrees who had returned to school for master's degrees. During several planning meetings with Silver that spring, Ford suggested that these nurses, because of their public health experience, would be most likely to function well in independent settings. In August of that year they began the program with a single student, Sue Stearly.

Stearly had just completed work on her master's degree after working both on hospital wards and in public health. Silver recalls, "She was a young, bubbly, energetic, pleasant, and ideal person—as a nurse or in any other kind of role." Because of her education and experience, she could have commanded a good salary working elsewhere, but Silver could offer her a stipend of only $400 a month, the money being supplied by the University's research committee. "I happened to be chairman of the committee," admits Silver in explaining how the financing became available.

The pediatrics department at the School of Medicine offered its tacit support to the program, but the School of Nursing, despite Ford's involvement, still seemed resistant to the idea. "I think it was justifiable resistance," concedes Silver. "The idea was new. We were trying to alter a role. I was a doctor trying to change the profession of nursing. They had to be conservative in what they allowed us to do."

Judith Igoe believes that part of the resistance was because for years nursing educators had been trying to establish the role of the nurse as a professional concerned with total care of the patient. "They were working for years to show that nursing can be more than looking to see that someone's heart is beating properly," states Igoe. "Simply handing a nurse a few of the doctor's tools was not going to improve health care in this country."

Silver's concept of the nurse practitioner, of course, went beyond that. There were no formal classes. Each morning Stearly would appear at Silver's office for instruction. They spent as much time as they felt they needed on specific subjects, then went on to something else. Sometimes they stayed in the office. Other times they visited different departments within the School of Medicine or at Colorado General Hospital across the street. Silver had taught medical students as well as residents, so knew what went into the training of pediatricians. But often he felt Stearly needed to learn something about a specific specialty—such as ear, nose, and throat (ENT)—so he would call a specialist in that area and arrange for her to have an appointment. "It was very unstructured," he says, "and that was probably one of the strongest things about the program. It allowed her to participate in developing her own educational experience."

On the first day, Silver asked Stearly, "Have you ever used a stethoscope?"

"Yes," responded Stearly. "I've listened to fetal hearts and taken blood pressure readings."

"Have your ever listened to the heart or lungs of an individual?"

"No."

Silver admits that even if she had done that, Stearly probably would not have admitted it, because such practices were not part of what constituted "nursing" in the traditional sense. That day he took her to the nursery and had her listen to the heart of an infant and describe what she heard. He then explained the meaning of the sounds heard through the stethoscope.

Stearly also helped mold her own program. One day she returned from a visit to the department of audiology to announce that she had arranged to spend four more sessions in that department. Considering the limited time available, Silver thought that much time seemed excessive, but decided that if it was important to her, she should follow her own instincts.

The time came for Stearly to end her training and put into practice what she learned. In mid-December, after four months, she appeared one morning at Silver's office and began to talk about leaving. At first he feared she was quitting the program. "I really got concerned," he said, "because I would be losing 100% of the program's student body." But what she really meant was that she was ready to go into practice. Stearly felt she had learned all she could in a school setting and would be able to progress better working with the public.

In searching for somewhere for her to practice, Silver and the new nurse practitioner felt she would be able to function best in a public health situation in a community with a definite need for more care. They identified Trinidad, Colorado, a town of 9,901 people 200 miles south of Denver, as a good location. Trinidad had five physicians; one a man in his seventies, another a state senator, and a third who had been brought in by the United Mine Workers, so there were few full-time, practicing physicians. A building on one of the school grounds that a janitor once lived in became vacant at that time, so it was converted into a clinic with the help of local volunteers. Stearly began practice there.

Silver was able to convince the local doctors that this new nurse practitioner was not coming into town to steal patients, but rather would add to the care they were giving patients. Many of the people in town attended a health department clinic, or if they got sick they called a doctor. Silver explained that this would still be happening, but the nurse practitioner would be screening patients, referring patients, and consulting with the doctors.

In the meantime, the second class of nurse practitioners, consisting of four nurses from the Denver Visiting Nurses Association, began training at the University of Colorado. Two of them, upon completing their training, located in an area near a housing project on the north side of the city that is isolated with railroad tracks on one side, a main highway on another, vacant lots on the third, and a slaughter house on the fourth. In the summer of 1966 they opened a health station in an apartment in this housing project. One afternoon a week, Silver acted as a consultant to the nurse practitioners; a physician with the health department was there on another day. The nurse practitioners demonstrated their capability in taking care of well children, determining their physical needs, and also managing some sick children without direct medical supervision. "They are very good at knowing their limits," explained Silver, "so can handle many of the minor illnesses ordinarily seen by doctors."

Silver continued to inform local members of the American Academy of Pediatrics about the progress of his plans, since he feared that if the pediatricians opposed his ideas they could effectively stop him, but the physicians mounted no challenge. Igoe explains why: "One thing that helped was that Dr. Silver's colleagues had a tremendous amount of respect for the way he conducted himself professionally as well as privately. Henry was not just a good doctor, but a well respected individual."

There are no precise definitions as to what comprises medicine and what comprises nursing; members of these two professions provide their own definitions partly by what they do in practice. At one end doctors diagnose and treat complicated illnesses; at the other end nurses support the patient and manage those illnesses. But in between, there is a lot of common ground.

One study made at the housing project indicated that the nurse practitioners were competent to handle 71% of all patients who walked into their clinic. Another 11% could be handled in the office if the nurse practitioner contacted the doctor by phone, relayed information and the symptoms, and obtained an opinion. (Doctors consult with each other in similar fashion.) The remainder had to be referred to a physician. Silver claims that numerous similar studies elsewhere seem to approximate this same 71% figure for the number of patients that a nurse practitioner can treat directly.

Another study, comparing how nurse practitioners and physicians identified problems, indicated that 84% of the time the two agreed completely on the "diagnosis" (although technically nurse practitioners do not diagnose). In 15% of the cases, the nurse practitioner and physician disagreed, but it made no difference in the treatment of the child. (For instance, one might have heard an innocent heart murmur and the other did not hear it, but no treatment was needed in either case.) In only two instances, according to Silver, were there disagreements of any significance. In one case the nurse said a child had a sore throat, and the physician later diagnosed meningitis. Later, the meningitis diagnosis was determined inaccurate. In another instance a nurse practitioner thought a child had bronchitis; it turned out to be pneumonia. Even in this case she did the proper thing: refer the sick child to a physician.

Dr. Silver explains that the 2% disagreement is probably less than would occur between two physicians for a simple reason: a nurse practitioner, in working with a physician, usually learns that particular physician's criteria in determining illnesses and tends to describe and define ailments according to those criteria. Nurse practitioners working with two or more physicians, however, sometimes have to report symptoms differently because of the way in which different physicians practice medicine.

Whether or not a nurse practitioner can "diagnose" is an issue because most state medical laws prevent a nurse from diagnosing or treating. Silver explains, "A nurse practitioner might say that there is a 'dullness in this part of the chest,' and if you ask her what does that suggest to you, she will reply pneumonia. But she does not write pneumonia on the chart. She writes the description of what she found. She doesn't say a patient has a strep throat, but rather he has a 'positive strep culture and red infected throat, nodes in his neck, and a fever.' But that's not a diagnosis." In Silver's office he keeps a list of synonyms for diagnosis and treatment. He says with a smile, "A nurse practitioner can *assess* or *evaluate,* but she doesn't diagnose; she can *manage* but she doesn't *treat.* What is most important is that what she does is done under supervision of a physician, and there's nothing new in that. Nurses on the wards in hospitals do the same, but on so-called 'standing orders' from the doctors. Many visiting nurse services actually have little books that nurses carry with them containing standing orders. 'This is what you do in this situation. This is what you do somewhere else.' In teaching nurse practitioners, we never went that far, but we always said, never do anything where there is any doubt. The worry I see about nurse practitioners is not that they may do too much, but rather that they may not do enough —and that usually is because of the policies of the physician they work with."

The acceptance of nurse practitioners by physicians outside Silver's circle of colleagues has lagged behind the public's acceptance of them. In another study done at the University of Colorado, 94% of patients accepted nurse practitioners. "The public was way ahead of us," states Silver. "They were already saying that nurse practitioners are good, and they're going to get better."

That study was completed in 1967 at a time Silver was encountering opposition from the nursing profession. He recalls, "I remember visiting the Children's Bureau in Washington and meeting with two or three physicians who said they thought it was a fine idea, then meeting with the nurses in the same office who indicated that this was a bad idea, that I was asking nurses to be junior doctors. I never thought of nurses as junior doctors; I thought of them as sharing health care for patients."

But not everyone within the nursing profession was opposed. When Silver gave presentations at nursing meetings and conventions, the senior nurses acted very cool toward him. But when he left the meeting and went outside, the younger nurses would stop him in the hall and say, "That's exactly what I went into nursing for."

Physicians' opposition has continued somewhat even after the nursing profession has finally embraced the concept of the practitioner. Silver believes that, almost without exception, anyone who has worked with a nurse practitioner, or has had any contact with one in a professional sense, has been enthusiastic about the usefulness of his or her professional training. Opposition at medical meetings where Silver presented his case usually came from someone who had no contact with nurse practitioners, frequently someone who felt financially threatened. When the issue of malpractice is raised, Silver states that he is not aware of a single malpractice suit initiated by a patient against a nurse practitioner. Malpractice rates as set by insurance companies reflect the low incidence of suits. A nurse can be insured against malpractice through the American Nurses Association for less than $100 compared to the thousands of dollars physicians must pay.

The acceptance of the nurse practitioner is evidenced by the fact that 200 institutions now offer training programs, and there are an estimated 8,000 to 12,000 nurse practitioner positions now filled. The profession is in the process of defining its own scope and limitations, since there presently is no certifying mechanism for nurse practitioners except for pediatric nurse practitioners who can obtain certification from the National Board of Pediatric Nurse Practitioners and Associates, the National Association of Pediatric Nurse Associates and Practitioners (NAPNAP), and from the American Academy of Pediatrics. Recently these organizations developed the national qualifying examination by which a nurse who has completed a formal course of study can be certified. This is the first examination that attempts to test the entry-level competence of the nurse practitioner. Silver believes that eventually a national organization will provide the same certification for nurse practitioners in all specialties.

Silver looks at the immediate future and suggests that, of all specialists, school nurse practitioners can make the greatest impact on health care in America by managing the treatment of children between ages 5 and 18. "It's because the children are so readily available. They're a captive population," he says. "The nurse practitioners can get at the kids and find things that essentially nobody assesses and manages well now: learning problems, behavioral difficulties, perceptual difficulties. We are doing more and more, but it has to be done in the school, since you can't always expect parents to bring their children to doctors' offices for problems that are not acute or serious. The school nurse practitioner could provide a tremendous amount of health care, both preventive and curative in school."

The value of the nurse practitioner is evident in one study done at the University of Colorado comparing the work of school nurses with that of school nurse practitioners. The study concluded that the school nurse practitioners, 1) tended to be more sharply focused and specific in their management of pupils' health problems; 2) excluded only about half as many pupils from school; 3) referred only about half as many pupils for consultation care or future evaluation; 4) were more likely to provide clear, specific advice to parents or excluded children, which resulted in more frequent compliance with school nurse practitioner recommendations.

In 1977 Dr. Silver wrote a letter to the White House recommending that the federal government establish a network of school nurse practitioner training programs throughout the U.S. in order to prepare a sufficient number to meet the unmet health needs of a large segment of America's child population. He wrote, "Since 1970, when we established the first school nurse practitioner training program in the U.S., we have been able to show that school nurse practitioners can give much of the health care and many of the health services required by school-age children. We have also demonstrated that schools can serve as one of the major settings where comprehensive primary and continuing care services are given, since the school is the one place where children between the ages of 5 and 18 years are regularly and readily accessible to obtain the health care they require."

He continued, "It should be emphasized that most 'regular' school nurses presently working in schools have had limited preparation as primary health care providers and are usually very restricted in what they are allowed to do. Regular school nurses need to become school nurse practitioners so they can have an expanded and more meaningful role as health providers. This can only be done by having them complete a course of study in a formal structured school nurse practitioner training program. . . .

"There is a need for a national project to establish at least 100 school nurse practitioner programs in all 50 states. This would be a practical and effective way of providing health care to school-age children regardless of their families' income, the place where they live, or the apathy their parents may have shown in taking them to health care providers. For a moderate expenditure of funds, we could achieve a marked increase in the quantity and quality of the health care and services that would be provided to the millions of children who are most in need of them. Effective utilization of specially prepared school nurse practitioners as primary health care providers would result in a major modification of the present health care system for children."

Thus far, the White House has shown no haste in responding with action for such a plan, but Silver has proven himself to be a man of patience as well as vision, and some day his dreams for such a training program for school nurse practitioners may come true.

Nurse practitioners will succeed or fail in the U.S. not on their ability to deliver care equal to the physician's, which is not their role, but on whether they can help make the entire health system work more efficiently. Health care is becoming increasingly more complex. The highly skilled physician finds himself torn between developing better patient relationships

53

and practicing medicine at a higher level of excellence. Furthermore, the health care system is going through a reorganization; the nurse practitioner is going to achieve increased acceptance as this reorganization takes place.

Judith Igoe, however, sounds one mild note of warning. She believes that, long before the nurse practitioner movement came along, nurses had specific activities that went beyond merely following the doctor's orders and taking patients' temperatures. Nurses took care of the total patient and helped that person through the stress of illnesses. But now she reports that recent studies of some nurse practitioners show them seeing patients at the rate of six an hour—in short, with the same frequency that many physicians rush through patients. "To me," says Igoe, "that eliminates the basic nursing activity of being the patient's advocate, working with people and showing them how they can improve their health. I would hate to see us spend less time in helping people take care of themselves."

Hopefully the nurse practitioner movement can be kept on the proper course to provide better care for more people. Utilizing nurse practitioners seems to be a logical route in providing health care, particularly at the school level. As we traveled the country to learn more about how we could improve the health of the pupils in Posen and Robbins, we discovered that several school systems already had begun to utilize nurse practitioners to provide better care for children. One of the most innovative is in Cambridge, Massachusetts. In that city, Dr. Philip J. Porter decided that the public health service should utilize the schools for a very logical reason. We shall examine that reason in the next chapter.

Part III: School Health in America

The Porter Principles—Cambridge

The children of Cambridge, Massachusetts, obtain health care under what might be termed a variation of "Willie Sutton's Law" (named after the famous bank robber). When we visited Dr. Philip J. Porter, director of that city's public health department, in his office on the fifth floor of Cambridge Hospital he explained to us, "It's like Willie Sutton's reply when asked why does he rob banks? 'That's where the money is.' Well, schools are where the children are."

He continued, "Being a pediatrician, where in the world would you look if you wanted to deliver health services?" Porter paused and waited for the obvious answer, then supplied it himself: "Well, the place that hits you right square in the face is in the schools."

Porter was stating a principle we also heard espoused by Dr. Charles U. Lowe, special assistant for child health affairs at the Department of Health, Education, and Welfare. Lowe phrased it slightly differently: "The schools tend to aggregate children, therefore bringing one provider to the aggregation is considerably more parsimonious of resources than having the provider sit in an office somewhere and, one by one, the children go to him." Thus, Willie Sutton's Law. Of course, Lowe had visited Cambridge, too, and came back to Washington praising it as one of the most exciting new health experiments in America.

Porter has totally restructured that city's public health program à la Willie Sutton. Cambridge is the home of Harvard University. In addition to this prestigious institution, however, Cambridge also includes public housing, ghetto apartments, and poverty similar to that found in almost any of our major cities.

When we were looking for models after which we could pattern the school health program in Posen-Robbins, Cambridge was the first place we visited. (We also visited Hartford, Connecticut, and Galveston, Texas, described in following chapters.) In Cambridge, Porter has replaced the traditional system of school nurses and school doctors with a staff of 15 pediatric nurse practitioners who work in clinics established in four of Cambridge's public schools as well as one in a municipal building adjacent to a school. In doing so, he has improved the level of health care within the city, while also lifting a burden from the shoulders of its physicians. Porter states, "When I used to go to my friends and ask, 'Would you like to be a school doctor in Cambridge,' they looked at me as if I had lost my mind. Nobody wanted that position."

Modern physicians dislike the role of school physician because of the episodic nature of the patient contact and thus, the lack of continuity of care. The tasks are often routine and seem to be an inefficient use of physician time. It also may be a financial waste to the patient, who may be able to obtain routine care less expensively from a different kind of health professional—if that health professional is available. In making that professional available, Porter raised the health consciousness of Cambridge families and showed how children throughout the country can have their health needs provided for at much lower cost.

Raised in Buffalo, New York, Philip Porter attended the University of Pennsylvania Medical School, trained at the Massachusetts General Hospital, spent time with the Air Force in Texas before returning to the Boston area in the sixties to work as a research fellow exploring infectious diseases in the Channing Research Laboratory at the Boston City Hospital.

In 1965 he joined the staff of what was then called Cambridge City Hospital; it is now the Cambridge Hospital. He admits, "After a period of time, we dropped 'City' from our title as a means of softening our image as the place in the community where only poor people went to get care."

In 1965 Porter encountered what he describes as chaos: "When I arrived, I worked mainly in the emergency ward taking care of the great volume of children who came in for episodic care because of illness or accident. We were so busy doing that, we rarely had time to consider longitudinal care. I thought, hopefully, there were some programs for this. But there weren't, because the same children kept bouncing back all the time."

Cambridge was not without health programs for children. In fact, it was over-programmed: well-baby clinics, school health programs, Head Start clinics, high school physical examination programs, as well as clinics at Cambridge Hospital and other hospitals in Greater Boston. "Care was totally fragmented," explains Porter. "Mothers sometimes had children in four different programs and spent all their time running from one to the other."

Health problems in the area were accentuated by the presence of a minority group, somewhat unique in its identity but with problems that are far from unique. Cambridge is a city of 100,361 people located across the Charles River from Boston and indistinguishable, at least to out-of-towners, from that larger city. One of the main Cambridge minority groups is Portuguese, approximately 10,000 of them live in Cambridge. More precisely this minority group is not merely Portuguese, but it is composed of people from the Portuguese Azores islands—and, more specifically, people from the island of San Miguel. Families from that island first arrived in New England several generations ago to work as fishermen in coastal towns such as New Bedford. Then, as the fishing industry stagnated, they drifted into the Boston area to obtain factory jobs. They settled first in Cambridge because of the availability of relatively low-cost apartment housing.

In the familiar pattern of ethnic settlement, new families followed old friends and relatives (sometimes illegally) swelling Cambridge's Portuguese population. After earning some money, the more industrious among this population moved to the next community of Somerville where they could buy homes. But most of Cambridge's shifting Portuguese population is first generation, still struggling with the language and strange ways of the New World. They are crowded into one section of town.

"Sociologically, Cambridge is two different cities," explains Porter. "If you dropped a perpendicular through Central Square, you would divide the city into West Cambridge and East Cambridge. West Cambridge is Harvard, Radcliffe; a fairly well-to-do, educated, and sophisticated community. East Cambridge is blue-collar, low-income; has a high rate of problems and includes the Portuguese community, a community obviously in need." All the problems one associates with the blacks of Chicago's west side, the Puerto Ricans of New York's Spanish Harlem, and the Chicanos of California's San Joaquin Valley are

58

visited upon the Portuguese of Cambridge. This is particularly true in terms of health care.

The people of West Cambridge visit private physicians. Harvard and MIT provide their own medical services for students, as well as community families. Many physicians live in West Cambridge because—in still another variation of Willie Sutton's Law—that's where the private patients are. They also are attracted by the presence of both Harvard Medical School and Massachusetts General Hospital across the Charles River. East Cambridge, however, is medically underpopulated. When Porter first arrived in 1965, he found 11 general practitioners in East Cambridge. Their median age was 59 and, he adds, "No young physicians were moving in. It's not unlike the history of any other inner city—Chicago, New York, Cleveland. Relatively few practicing physicians live in the inner city."

As a result, the emergency ward at Cambridge Hospital became "general practitioner" for the community. According to Porter: "People were using the emergency ward for bee bites, skinned knees, colds, and you simply knew there had to be a better way to do it. Emergency wards are great when you are in an automobile accident or break a leg, but they are not terribly good if you have a child who always suffers from a cold. With physicians rotating through, a family never gets to see the same doctor, so they get 50 different answers to the same questions. Nobody is able to take time to look at the child's total health picture, or the family's total health picture. It was like papering over a crack in the wall. Unless you deal with the underlying problem, the crack will always show through."

By analyzing the addresses on emergency ward slips, Porter learned that most patients using emergency services lived in East Cambridge, in and around the low-income housing projects. After being appointed director for maternal and child health in Cambridge in 1968, he decided to apply Willie Sutton's Law and try to provide care for these patients through the most highly visible and centrally located organization in the communities of greatest need: the school system.

"In 1968 the city of Cambridge had a school building campaign," says Porter. "Their schools had gotten old, and the city planned to build new ones. The superintendent let me work with the architects and we drew in functional health suites in each new unit."

Thus, the Cambridge school health system was organized on what might be called the Five Porter Principles.

"The first principle," Porter explained to us during our visit, "was to put all the public programs for child health in one administrative framework. This enables you to develop continuing comprehensive programs so that one child does not get 50 shots while another child gets zero shots. They get the right number. The only way to accomplish that is to have a single administrative cover: one person making sure the services are age-appropriate and that everyone eligible gets them.

"Since the 1930s, in most cities," he continues, "a series of child health programs have developed. Municipalities pay for them like other city services. Child health services have developed like topsy over 45 years and have become fragmented, disorganized, and end up separating the sick child in the hospital from the well child in school. But it's the same child at different times in his life. These are traditional public health services, but when you look at these programs critically, you might not be so happy at what they are providing in terms of the needs of today's children. They are limited in scope. Needs change, times change, and programs have to change as well. What often happens is that needs change, times change, but programs remain the same."

So the first Porter Principle became: *Centralize Administrative Functions.*

"The second principle," Porter continues, "is that you can centralize the administration, but if you put all these services in one place you will cause a great number of people serious inconvenience. You can create a setting that is impossible to reach. This is particularly true if you put your services in an already crowded hospital. People who have to travel to a centralized service also may avoid doing so because they don't have a car, don't want to spend money to take public transportation, or they simply don't want to bother. This is particularly true with preventive services when no one is seriously ill.

"But perhaps a more important reason for avoiding hospitals in the delivery of these services is cost. Hospitals are very costly places, even for routine care. They charge you simply for stepping across their threshold, so in practice you ought to use hospitals only for costly medical problems. If you have a cold, the emergency ward of Massachusetts General is not the place to go. You won't necessarily get better treatment there, but you will get a higher bill.

"A less expensive place from where care can be dispensed—again following Willie Sutton's Law—is in the schools. For the most part they are already built, already located in the neighborhoods; children attend them and parents can get to them easily. They are the logical places in which to dispense low-cost treatment for children."

The second Porter Principle, following this logic, is: *Don't Dispense in a High-Cost Area Services That Can Be Delivered More Cheaply Elsewhere.*

"The third principle," says Porter, "revolves around a developing trend in medicine that recognizes that not all the functions performed by physicians one and two generations ago need be performed by them today. Medicine has changed rapidly since World War II, and the former general practitioners who dispensed aspirins and cough syrup and rode to their patients' homes via horse and buggies and later Model T Fords, have disappeared along with those modes of transportation. They have been replaced by modern physicians with much more specialized training, who themselves have been compartmentalized into increasingly sophisticated disciplines. A neurologist does not make house calls, because he needs a cadre of assistants and associates in an expensively equipped arena in order to perform the complicated task he does so well.

"This era of medical specialization has left a vacuum in health care that can be filled by health professionals who do not have M.D. degrees, but who can function ably under the supervision of a physician. In Cambridge, we've chosen nurse practitioners, registered nurses who have undergone additional training so that they can perform many of the routine, but necessary medical tasks that were once the prerogatives of general practitioners.

"These nurse practitioners form the first line of entry into the total pediatric care system here. The second line is the physician, who sees more seriously ill patients referred to him by the nurse practitioner. The third line is the specialist, or specialist hospital, where the most seriously ill patients can get intensive care or specialist treatment."

Porter concludes: "Children are basically healthy, and if you try to keep some of society's problems off their backs, they will continue to be generally healthy, with the exception of minor respiratory illnesses. Most of these complaints can be managed by a nurse practitioner with the supervision of a pediatrician."

The third Porter Principle, thus, is: *Use the Simplest Means To Provide the Simplest Care, and Use Complicated Means Only for Complicated Care.*

"The fourth principle involves financing," continues Porter. "Once having centralized the administration, decentralized the service, and agreed to use pediatric nurse practitioners to be the backbone of the delivery system, the next need was for money to finance the program. In Cambridge's case, the money had been available since the mid-thirties, going into school health and well-baby clinics. It was simply a matter of reallocating existing monies to support new programs that meet existing needs."

The fourth Porter Principle, therefore, is: *Place Your Money Where Your Needs Are.*

"The fifth and final principle," summarizes Porter, "is measuring your achievements. Having applied the first four principles, have you been able to improve the bottom line figures related to the health of the people you serve?

"In Cambridge, the most obvious indication of success was at the emergency ward, where in 1965, 70% of the children were brought there for medically inappropriate reasons. Since it was the only place to go, it was appropriate, but if there is somewhere else available, you should not go to the emergency ward with a cold or diaper rash. After we got our school-based health program into effect, 'inappropriate' use of emergency ward services by Cambridge patients was cut in half, to 35%. No similar change in the pattern of emergency ward utilization occurred among residents of neighboring Somerville, not served by a similar program."

Porter also offers other statistical examples of success. In terms of immunization, only 55% of children entering school in 1965 were immunized; the immunization rate a decade later rose to 98%. The frequency of lead poisoning dropped from 7% to one half of 1%. The penetration of the program is such that close to 95% of all children in the area served by the program are covered by it. This area covers East Cambridge, which includes 50% of all children in Cambridge. Incidences of iron deficiency anemia also have been reduced significantly: From 16% to 4% in one- to two-year-olds.

Perhaps another consideration, not so easily measured statistically, has been the effect on the medical education of the Harvard Medical School students and house officers from Massachusetts General Hospital who rotate through Cambridge Hospital. "We have about 25 pediatricians in training coming through every year and 50 medical students," says Porter, "and they all rub up against this program and have an opportunity to see what primary care for pediatrics can be."

The fifth, and final, Porter Principle, might be said to be: *The Success of Your Program Should Be Documented.*

Thus far, the Cambridge school health program not only has proved its own success but has served as a model for others interested in providing better health care for children within the school system, including those from Posen-Robbins School District 143½.

In initiating his program, Porter first approached the school nurses then working in the Cambridge schools and asked if they would like to upgrade their skills by attending classes to become pediatric nurse practitioners. Most were nearing retirement and had little interest in change. At the same time, very few young persons were becoming school nurses. According to Porter, "The job of school nurse wasn't that attractive for bright young people coming out of nursing school. They wanted to be where the action was, and that wasn't in the basement of a school."

He retained some of the school nurses already in the system, but began rewriting job descriptions for those who eventually would be hired as their replacements. His goal for each school was to have two or three nurse practitioners, operating in group practice with a social worker. The nurse practitioners would have clinical responsibilities for examining children, screening their illnesses, and immunizing them. They also would visit homes in the neighborhood to talk to parents. Their goal would be to learn how many children were in each family and what problems they had. In addition, they were expected to work with the teachers in the school to learn about problem children: the ones who had a learning disability or behavioral problems. Only if they could identify children with solvable problems could they help them.

Typical among the schools in East Cambridge is the Harrington School, bordering on the Portuguese community and near Roosevelt Towers, a public housing project. In 1973, Cindy Wilke arrived at Harrington. Born in Rochester, New York, she attended nursing school there and worked in Johns Hopkins Hospital in Baltimore before accepting a post at Massachusetts General Hospital in Boston. She later became head nurse on the obstetrical floor at Cambridge Hospital where Porter recruited her to take the 17-week course at Northeastern University to become a pediatric nurse practitioner. She soon began practicing in that capacity at Harrington School.

The health center at Harrington School occupies a suite of rooms across the hall from the master's office. (Master is the term by which principals are referred to in much of New England.) Few of the Cambridge masters showed much enthusiasm for the new health centers crowding into their educational facilities and staffed by energetic young nurses who didn't seem to know their place in the complicated order of the school. Cindy Wilke explains, "When I first came here there was a school nurse who performed many functions for the master; however, I felt my job was to take care of the children, not the master."

Antagonisms developed early between the administration and the new health professionals at the center. The administration was insistent on knowing who the "school nurse" was. The nurse practitioners made up a duty roster identifying a different one of them as "school nurse" on succeeding weeks. After that, relationships began to improve.

"We began going out of our way to be accommodating," admitted Wilke. She adds, "An essential part of being situated within the school is to be sensitive to the needs of the teachers as well as the administration. We really are intruding sometimes. There are a lot of people coming and going as a result of our being here."

This was because the school health program in Cambridge was designed not merely to provide health care for children attending kindergarten to eighth grade, but it also encompassed other age groups, particularly preschool children and sometimes adolescents. The goal of Porter's program was not merely to cure problems once the children entered school, but to correct them *before* entry, and hopefully to prevent them altogether. This goal could be accomplished only if those families who would benefit from the service would learn of it five years before their child entered kindergarten.

A good deal of the success of the Cambridge school health project comes from its outreach into the community, which is accomplished in a number of ways. Half of Cambridge mothers deliver their babies in various hospitals scattered throughout Greater Boston, but eventually their birth certificates are processed through City Hall. Porter receives a copy of these certificates and alerts a nurse practitioner.

"We then make a home visit," explains Wilke. "The purpose is to say, 'Here we are. Have you thought about pediatric care for your child?'" While in the home, they also inquire about any older brothers and sisters. The same principle operates in reverse when a child from a new family enrolls in a Cambridge school served by the program. "Do you have any younger brothers or sisters at home?" the receiving nurse practitioner will ask.

Other sources of referral are emergency ward records, which

are sorted geographically. The nurse practitioners receive reports of emergency ward visits by patients, then contact them to find if the temperature is down and if the parents are giving the prescribed medication. Wilke says, "It's a good way of picking up patients who do not use the center but use the emergency ward inappropriately. This has been one of the main ways in which we have been able to cut down use of the emergency ward."

Suspicious of the system at first, teachers and administrators soon realized that the general health of Harrington students was improved by the presence of the three nurse practitioners in the building. Better relationships with the teachers also have occurred, Wilke reports. "Over the years we have developed more of a rapport with the teachers just by knocking on their doors and saying, 'Hi, I'm Cindy. How are things going? If you have any problems, drop by.' We also have nurse/teacher conferences. It's been slow and gradual to have some kind of input into health education. We get invited to do a bit more each year. We are gradually getting our feet in the door.

"If teachers have concern as to the vision or hearing of one of their students, we know places to refer them. There is so much red tape in the school system when you refer children for evaluation, but we often know a faster and better way to accomplish what is needed. We also counsel parents of preschoolers so problems do not come up, such as with teeth that never have been seen by a dentist until sixth grade when a child comes in with big abscesses. Many preventive services are being rendered before they become problems."

But so far only half the children within the Cambridge school system fall under the school health program. Health centers are established in only four of Cambridge's nine schools. Some of the children in schools with school health centers may receive care from private physicians rather than from the clinic. "There is somewhat of a differentiation between children who are followed regularly here for health care," admits Wilke. "We do more for them than the child who goes to a private doctor, because we do not want to intrude on a private practice. Health records are marked as to whether or not they are a clinic patient. If so, we might go ahead and do a throat culture. If not, we would be more inclined to call the mother and say her child should see a doctor."

Cambridge, Massachusetts, provided us with a unique model for our school health program, but we still had much more to learn when we next visited Hartford, Connecticut.

A Health Program for Hartford

Several years ago the Children's Television Workshop, producers of "Sesame Street," approached the school system in Hartford, Connecticut, with a proposal for an experimental public service advertising project. The TV people wanted to air a series of health-oriented commercials in the Hartford area aimed at increasing the immunization level of children in that city. The school administrators tried to discourage the "Sesame Street" producers, pointing out that Hartford already had a high immunization rate for its children, nearly 90%.

Nevertheless, Children's Television Workshop people wanted to proceed, mainly because of the demographic characteristics of the city. Hartford was neither so large to make it difficult to handle the additional immunizations the campaign supposedly would generate, nor so small that the numbers immunized would seem statistically unimpressive. They hoped to get 5,000 children immunized, both school-age children and preschoolers. Finally, after two months of planning, the TV campaign began and children were exhorted, via "Sesame Street," to have their parents take them to public health clinics for immunization shots.

The results proved disappointing. Only 650 children appeared for immunization. And the campaign had one negative factor, according to Joseph Constantine, director of guidance and health services for the Hartford schools: it raised anxiety levels among parents whose children already were immunized. "Hartford has a history of providing health services for its school children," he reported. "We're probably one of the few school systems in the country—and definitely in Connecticut—that does immunizations routinely. We were simply a poor choice for the TV campaign."

Nevertheless, even Constantine readily admitted that, like most other school systems, Hartford was not doing everything it could to provide maximum health care for its children. In Hartford, nurses in the school system gave immunizations, while outside physicians gave physicals to the children. Routine hearing and vision screening identified health problems. But as is the case elsewhere, once having pinpointed problems, the school system did little to alleviate them or to determine if the children's parents sought further care.

Typically, each school had its school nurse, but he or she had little authority to act. Judy Lewis of the University of Connecticut Health Center stated what had become a familiar theme to us: "Traditionally, school nurses do what they're supposed to do. In the inner-city schools, they face different and difficult problems. They have teachers and parents bringing problems to them that they can't do much about. They don't even have a nurse's aide at most schools. One nurse might have responsibility for 800 children with all the paperwork necessitated by that many children." Lewis indicated that providing adequate medical care for many children in Hartford seemed an impossible task—at least until a few years ago.

She added, "A lot of people put down school nurses because they supposedly have soft jobs and don't want to do anything. But school nurses don't have the skills to do a lot of things, and furthermore, may not be sanctioned to do them." Yet some people in Hartford, particularly at the University of Connecticut Health Service where Dr. Margaretta E. Patterson was director of pediatrics, were aware of both the problems and the potential for health care in the Hartford school system. Patterson thought that the school nurse had much more potential than previously realized and that she also could provide a "linkage" between the health needs of children and their educational needs, particularly in the inner city.

"Several things are happening in this country," Patterson told us during our visit to Hartford, "and one of them is that many children are not getting services, and probably the only way these services can be given is in school. Their total exposure to health care is through a school nurse.

"We started looking at why they didn't get care and it turned out that most of these overlooked children—and Silver in Colorado estimates that there are between seven and eight million of them in this country—lack health care not just because they're poor. Actually, all the poor children in this city can have care if they want it. It's for many other reasons."

Patterson outlined some of them, "It's because the families can't get to the doctor; they lack transportation; or, they don't know how to get there, maybe partly because they don't talk the language. Just getting your child into the care system is difficult. The care is *here,* but the people are over *there,* and they don't know how to get from here to there.

"You can have outreach programs, but most outreach programs have been miserable failures, expensive ones at that. But here is your outreach program." Patterson waved her hand around her. We had been talking to her at one of the Hartford schools. "The *school* is your outreach program. Every child has to come to school. And the school nurse knows every child and is the one person in that child's life who is best able to provide entry into the health care system."

It seems we had encountered, once more, Willie Sutton's Law.

Hartford, Connecticut, has problems within its inner city identical to those in many inner cities throughout the U.S., although with a flavor somewhat unique. The city has 24 elementary schools, two middle schools, and three high schools. The school population is tremendously mobile, and it is not unusual for one child in fourth or fifth grade to have attended eight or nine different schools, all within the same school system. Forty percent of the children come from families on welfare. Certain schools have even higher than average percentages of welfare families. At the Hooker School, located near the Charter Oak Terrace public housing project, 80% of the families receive welfare checks.

The greatest increase among the inner city population has been among the Puerto Ricans. Some of them arrived in Hartford directly from the island to join families and friends; others moved there from New York City. These often impoverished families are attracted to Hartford by the availability of migrant farm work in the rural areas surrounding the city. The central Connecticut valley is a large farming area, particularly for tobacco used to make the outside wrappings for cigars. In the Hooker school, 65% of the students are Puerto Rican, 30% are black, and 5% are white.

The health care provided for these children, and the children of other Hartford inner-city neighborhoods, was mostly hit-and-miss. These poor people obtained medical care sometimes from the department of health and sometimes from the University of Connecticut Medical School's pediatrics department.

68

Several hospitals also provided ambulatory care; health clinics functioned in a few of the more destitute neighborhoods. There also were a few private physicians. Connecticut has many doctors to serve its population, but typically those doctors do not practice within the inner cities. As a result, many of the people with medical problems had to circulate from one health center to another, with little continuity of care. Medical personnel within the community recognized existing problems but did not know how to solve them.

Among the concerned institutions was the University of Connecticut. According to Judy Lewis: "We were surprised at the amount of illness among the school children. Everybody says that school-age kids are basically healthy. That may be true if you live in an area where you have a lot of services, those services are accessible, and people understand how to use them. But it's not true in the inner city.

"It's questionable how much health education ever goes on, because you continually tell children certain things about hygiene and health care, yet they often don't get any treatment for their problems. This is particularly true in the area of dental hygiene. You clean their teeth and identify cavities, but the cavities never get filled. There is no incentive to change behavior at all.

"Even if a parent follows through on a referral, a lot of things may happen during that interaction. There may be some psychological barrier between parent and the facility. The parents may not like the health person who sees them, or they don't understand the instructions, so their child does not get the benefit of the recommended care. But most damaging, the people back at the school referring the family to the physician never realized this. There was no follow-up. If the child didn't get treatment, nine times out of 10 the school would not find out about it. If it did, it would only be by accident, when a nurse looked through the file folder, saw the referral, and saw no entry since then. Only then would she realize the child had not received care."

The University of Connecticut decided to take one school within the inner city and attempt to improve its health care. In selecting the school, the University determined that first, it needed to be easily identifiable as needing health services. Second, it had to have no access to regular health services. Finally, there needed to be an acceptance on the part of the school staff to take part in such a project.

Hooker School was willing to serve as a project model; however, when the proposal to increase health services was brought to the school system administration, the administrators opposed the project for three reasons. First, bringing a health service of this nature into the school and making it fully operational would be burdensome administratively. Second, it would raise expectations of people using the service who would expect the project to continue *ad infinitum*, which might not be possible financially. (The Robert Wood Johnson Foundation was planning to fund the project for only the first three years.) Third, there would be pressure on the school system to continue the program, which might mean that health services eventually would have to compete with the educational program for available money within the budget.

As a result, when the proposal came before the board of education, the recommendation by the administration was that it not be approved. However, Lewis and Patterson had done their political homework by contacting board members in advance and pointing out the positive aspects of the program. The board decided to ignore the administration's recommendations and approved the project by a strong majority.

To add balance to the school health project, its directors decided to expand by adding a school in suburban Bloomfield. So the overall project became one urban and one suburban model. In addition, schools were identified in Bloomfield and Hartford in which project staff would document routine health services and compare those services to health programs in the model schools.

When we first visited the Hartford, Connecticut, project in September, 1975, to see if the experience gained from that project might give us some ideas applicable to our own project in Posen and Robbins, we found that the Hartford project had barely begun. We stopped only a short time on that first visit because there was not yet that much to see, but we did find the Hartford project different from what we had encountered in Cambridge only one day earlier.

Those providing health care in the school system in Cambridge had been connected to the hospital and the department of health, but they chose to provide their services in a school setting. In Hartford, however, all the staff members were employees of the board of education. The only two exceptions were the dentists and the pediatricians, who for liability reasons were paid through the University of Connecticut.

The medical services began in the fall of 1975, with the first clinic located in a pair of joined mobile homes on the playground behind Hooker School. The dental component did not begin operation until February, 1976. "We started slowly," admitted Lewis when we saw her on another visit to Hartford nearly one year later. By that time the health unit was fully operational. "We didn't want to hit the people of the community with a whole bunch of new ideas and not deliver, because traditionally, people in low-income groups get used." In comparison to the typical clinic in many cities that size, which often have massive waiting rooms with dozens of people coming and going, the simple unit behind Hooker School provided a nonthreatening environment. "Nobody feels uncomfortable coming here," said Lewis, "especially after they have had contact and established a relationship."

The two model programs were totally different. The one at Hooker School in the inner city provided primary health and dental care to all children in the school. In Bloomfield, where the parents have more money and often utilize private physicians, the focus was more on identifying problems and making referrals rather than getting involved in treatment of those problems. There also was a stronger emphasis on the educational needs of the children.

One of the first steps taken at Bloomfield was to upgrade the skills of the regular school nurse to those of a nurse practitioner. In addition, a series of classes for nurses in all the schools was begun.

"In this system [Hartford] the school nurse had been almost like the lowest person on the totem pole," said Lewis. "Nobody paid any attention to her. They hardly considered her a professional. With this training, she became *the* health professional in the school. I can't understand how all these years we had these nurses sitting around usually doing nothing. This was a mammoth untapped resource."

When the move was made to increase the responsibilities of the school nurse, surprisingly little opposition arose from pediatricians. The school nurses in their new roles were doing the sort of tasks that doctors normally disliked anyway: basic diagnosis and all the paperwork.

The Hooker School project became an immediate success, and in its first year the health team had contact with 91% of the children in the school. With the unit established, the two nurse practitioners now discover that they get a lot of child-initiated referrals. If children have sore throats, they come in expecting a throat culture. If they have earaches, they similarly appear for treatment. Sometimes they come in with questions about minor irritations. "It can be quite bothersome at times," admits nurse Pat Suarez, "but it's still a joy to know that you've made an impact on those children."

As for the success of the program, the absence rates for children with certain clinical conditions is low. "The one statistic that particularly stands out in my mind," states Joseph Constantine, "was that last year there was not one case of a ruptured eardrum, compared to the previous year when there were about half a dozen cases—the result of ear infections not being treated in time."

Another intangible is that the school children at Hooker are learning how to become better health consumers, which will make them better patients in their adult lives, and in turn will cause them to seek better health care for their children, thus breaking the chain of medical neglect from one generation to another.

"What we have done," says Constantine, "is to introduce the youngster and the family into the mainstream of health services. A much larger percentage of youngsters now get into hospitals for treatment with this kind of arrangement compared to those in other schools where the nurse makes a referral and too often it ends at that point. The program thus serves as a catalyst for better health care."

If good medical care had been difficult for the people living in the neighborhood around Hooker School to obtain before establishment of the school health unit, dental care was even more difficult. One reason was financial. "The cost of certain dental treatments is prohibitive to the low-income population," admits Dr. Alan Hindin, one of two dentists attached to the unit at Hooker. "You are dealing with 25% of their yearly income."

But even when financing is possible, it does not follow that good care becomes available. As it was with the physicians, despite a high ratio of dentists per population within the Hartford area, only a few dentists work in the inner city. Most Hartford dentists don't take welfare patients, especially Spanish-speaking ones. Cavities rarely get filled. The most frequent form of primary care for people with dental problems occurs at emergency room clinics—where the teeth get pulled. That's one of the few dental treatments where it is easy to obtain reimbursement from the welfare department.

Before coming to Hartford, Hindin served as a dentist in the U.S. Army, working at an installation in Columbia, South Carolina, that included in its population many people from the Appalachian area who never had seen a dentist during the first two decades of their lives. He saw what he described as extensive oral breakdown.

Hindin comments: "The attitude of these people was, 'Well, my grandfather had dentures, my father had dentures, so it's all right for me.' Breaking that chain poses a very difficult educational problem. Men don't come into the Army to be told their whole lifestyle needs change; they come in to put in their two years and go back home. There is only so much you can do in a few hours of talking to people. If you could start talking to them at the elementary school level, maybe you wouldn't see such poor teeth later in their lives."

While physicians have begun to expand their practices, and extend their services by use of nurse practitioners, physician's assistants, health associates, and other paraprofessionals, this movement has not yet spread to the dentists' ranks. According to Hindin: "The use of paraprofessionals in dentistry in the U.S. is way behind times. The resistance of the professional dental associations toward new ideas has dictated to us what tomorrow *will* be, rather than what it *can* be, and I think it's basically a question of security."

He adds, "When we first come out of dental school, we often are technique-oriented. We worry less about whether the patient is better than we worry if the technique is good. Dentists like to feel they are using modern techniques, but we're not as modern as we could be when it comes to providing treatment for as many people as possible. We have to step back and recognize that lesser-trained people can do things we can do on a technical level merely with technical training—not with four years of college, four years of dental school, and a year or two of residency.

"I've been involved politically in trying to generate the equivalent of nurse practitioners in dentistry. Such dental assistants have been trained quite successfully around the country on research grants, but we have been prevented from using them by state boards of examiners. The Forsythe Dental Center in Boston several years ago was a classic example. They had a beautiful program running using dental hygienists as nurse practitioners under close supervision. They were performing dental techniques successfully, but the state board in Massachusetts closed them down. Dr. DiPagio's program in Virginia was similar, but the state board again prevented the development of what would have been an innovative move toward providing dental care at a lower price to more people. So the use of dental nurse practitioners is out of the question right now in the U.S., unless there are some sweeping rule changes in the government structure.

"The limit of treatment that the current breed of dental hygienists provide usually includes taking x rays and cleaning teeth. Compared with regular medicine, the dental assistants have moved up from being orderlies to being licensed practical nurses. There is no way yet they can move up to the equivalent of registered nurses, physician's assistants, or nurse practitioners. They can go as high as hygienists, but no higher unless they become dentists, which is like asking the nurse to become a physician in order to do stitches. Physician's assistants do stitches and put on casts. They perform such tasks because it makes it more practical to deliver lower-cost medical care. As expensive as medical care is today, imagine how much it would cost if physicians put on all the casts, did all the stitches, did all the x rays, and carried all the bed pans. But that's the way many dentists still operate."

Hooker School did have some minimal dental care for its children prior to the establishment of the new health unit. The school building contained one room equipped with a dental chair, but the equipment was not adequate for good restorative work. About all the dentist could do was examine teeth and determine that they were decayed. As with medical problems similarly identified, there was no follow-up.

But the school (again following Willie Sutton's Law) would seem to be the ideal place to provide dental treatment. Hindin agrees. "What we have here is a 'waiting room' filled with 800 children, all of whom need treatment. We can tailor our whole process to the needs of the patient rather than the needs of the office."

By the "needs of the office" Hindin means the need for the dentist to schedule himself properly throughout the business day so that he does not waste time, which equates with money. Whereas the time the typical physician might spend with a patient is an average of five or 10 minutes, sometimes less, the dentist rarely spends less than a half hour with each patient, and often spends more. Each visit involving dental time is, in effect, a minor surgical procedure. If one patient fails to appear for an appointment—and inner-city people are notorious for missing appointments or cancelling them at the last minute —then the dentist has a large block of unproductive time that cannot be filled.

In the school setting, however, with those 800 potential patients sitting in classrooms less than a minute walk away, a missed appointment would cause less interruption in the scheduling of a dentist's day. "If a child is not here for an appointment," explains Lewis, "we simply call over to the main building and ask for another child as a substitute in that time slot."

Such flexibility in scheduling becomes particularly useful in dealing with the apprehensive child. Many children fear visiting the dentist's office with its strange looking machinery that whirrs and whines. They fear pain. Even more to the point, they fear the unknown. The dentist in private practice, faced by an apprehensive child, may attempt to calm that child's nerves, but sooner or later, within the time period scheduled for treatment, that child will have his tooth drilled or filled whether he likes it or not. And if the dentist does not want to force his technical procedures on the wary child, he may be forced to do so by the practical-minded parent standing nearby who knows he must pay whether or not treatment occurs. As a result, apprehensive children become even more apprehensive about future dental visits.

Hindin handles the apprehensive child at Hooker School simply by telling the child to watch and see how he works on other children. "We try to show children they are not trapped in a dental office," he states. He brings another child from the ever-present patient population in the school to the clinic and treats him while the apprehensive child watches. Sometimes the waiting child may be given some task to do involving the treatment of other children. Hindin occasionally hands a child a flashlight and asks him to look for cavities in someone else's mouth. "If the child sees a hole, he calls us over," says Hindin. "They usually spot something."

Children who have successfully "run the gauntlet" of the dentist chair come back to their classrooms and report what happened to them. At "show and tell" they proudly display their new plastic fillings. Their ability to withstand the rigors of the dental chair becomes a badge of courage that they wear proudly. Under such circumstances it is a rare individual who can resist peer pressure and continue to avoid proper dental treatment. Of 30 recent "problem" children, only three were not eager to come back to the dental unit. "Sometimes a child won't let me touch him, but he will come back and watch," says Hindin. "If it means three months of watching, that's okay. It doesn't cost us anything."

Because all the children in the school are constantly informing everybody else about what goes on in the dental unit, Hindin finds that he must practice honest dentistry; no tricks. This includes being open about Novocaine injections. "In dental school, we were taught to bring the syringe up under the chin, where the child couldn't see it—then *whammo!* But these are street kids, and they don't like being sneaked up on."

Respect for the child also carries over to respect for the teacher by arranging appointment schedules, when possible, so as not to disrupt classroom activities. If teachers feel the appointment interferes with an educational activity, they have the option of calling the unit and requesting a change of appointment for a child for dental or medical treatment. According to Lewis, "This was critical in gaining the support of the teachers and staff."

Modifications in the program occurred as Hindin and his colleague, Dr. Jack Levine, discovered the differences in providing care in a classroom setting compared to a normal office setting. When a cumbersome portable x ray machine broke down, Hindin and his two assistants, Elinor Norton and Angela Vona, discovered they actually could learn more with a routine screening in the classroom with tongue depressors and flashlights. If they saw something suspicious, the child could be brought into the office later for x rays on the larger machine. "Ellie and Angela tend to be more scrutinizing than I am sometimes," admits Hindin, "because they want to make sure they don't miss anything that I might find later. With the three of us giving examinations at the same time, we can run through a whole section of the school in a day-and-a-half."

Education also is an important function of the dental unit. At first, Hindin and Levine tried a structured teaching program provided by the dental association that utilized slides geared more to middle-class white children. "The kids here couldn't understand any of it," claims Hindin. "The slides talked about 'acid' eating the teeth. That term didn't work for children under the junior high level." He eventually replaced the presentation with slides showing children from Hooker School receiving dental treatment. The sight of their classmates being used as examples caused the children to pay closer attention to the dental hygiene message being offered them.

Although the dental program available at the Hooker School is unique in the U.S., such programs operate routinely in places such as Western Canada, New Zealand, and other parts of the world. In New Zealand, specially trained nurses do actual restorative work in the school setting. These countries use health extenders backed up by a dentist to deliver basic dental care. According to Hindin, studies indicate that these children have healthier teeth than American children even though the low-speed equipment being used is nowhere near as modern or efficient as that used in this country.

Lewis raises a basic philosophical question that is germane to the entire concept of medical treatment proposed in this book: "Providing health services as part of the school system is fine," she says, "but is that a function of the school? Should parents be dependent on the school for things they should provide themselves?" Lewis answers her own questions when she says, "There is a strong educational component here that nobody was initially aware of. I'm convinced that when we organize our health care in a setting where a child spends most of the day, where we can more easily determine their problems, and where we can have full access to them on a day-to-day basis so we can see that those problems get solved, we also will become more successful at educating them and keeping them in school."

She pauses. "Then the next question is: how do you make it financially possible for a program like this to exist in the schools?" That is a critical question and one that we will address later in this book.

Health on the Island—Galveston

Galveston is an island of 62,000 people on the Gulf coast of Texas. Residents refer to themselves as living, not in the city, but rather on "the Island." At the eastern end of the Island is the mammoth University of Texas Medical Branch, the oldest and largest medical school in Texas and, in the opinion of many, one of the better ones in the nation. Residents refer to it, on paper, as UTMB. In spoken conversation it is not the University, but rather "the Medical Branch." Within the Medical Branch's complex are seven hospitals. On staff are 685 physicians. The problem in Galveston was not the availability of medical services for its population, many of whom are low income, but rather the *utilization* of those services.

"There are plenty of doctors and clinics right where the people live," explains Dr. Philip Nader, medical director of school health services at the Galveston Independent School District, "but they weren't being utilized. So the need here in Galveston was not to provide health services, because there were adequate health services in the community. The need was to facilitate *access* to those services. Since the children—and through them, their families—were in the schools, we chose that as the point of access."

The Galveston Independent School District (GISD) serves about 11,000 children, half of them using the Medical Branch as their source of health care, the other half going to private physicians. These children attend one duo-campus high school, four middle schools, and nine elementary schools. The ethnic blend of Galveston includes three major groups: 42% black, 35% Anglo-American, and 23% Mexican-American. The socioeconomic distribution, according to one scale, lists 3% upper class,

2% upper-middle class, 36% lower-middle class, and 46% lower class.

When we visited Galveston in November, 1975, as part of our survey of school health programs, we recognized many similarities between the program there and the ones in Cambridge, Massachusetts, and Hartford, Connecticut. One difference, however, particularly compared with Cambridge, was that Galveston had better integrated its program into the school system. Another difference was that the nurse practitioners in Galveston did less diagnosis and treatment, perhaps because of the availability of so many physicians nearby. (Because of the University of Texas Medical Branch, the doctor/population ratio in Galveston is about 1 to 125, nearly 10 times greater than the national average.)

Nader was quite aware of the differenes between the Galveston program and that of Cambridge: "If you are in the health system, then you are somewhat distant from the educational system. If you are—as we are here—in the educational system, then you have some distance from the health system."

When we visited the school administration building, we talked with Mildred C. Williamson, coordinator of health services for GISD. "A lot of schools get someone in public health or a school nurse to do screening of vision or hearing. And maybe the physical education teachers take some heights and weights, but that's about it. You have to become much more involved in health if you are going to achieve our goal, which is to help the child know his own health needs and learn how to meet them by the time he graduates from high school. That's a big package."

Nader comments, "You must establish some kind of link between the schools and primary health care. You have the schools out here at Point A identifying problems, and you have the health care institution over here at Point B. But how do you get them together? One way to draw a line between points A and B is to hire home school agents to bridge the gap. Another way is to expand the school nurse's role. If you function like they do in Cambridge, the nurse may actually be delivering care. Not so here. We try to have our nurses become better problem identifiers. They become the main link."

The impetus for a new kind of school health program in Galveston dates back to the early 1970s. At that time GISD utilized a general practitioner as its school physician. She retired from school health at a time when the new superintendent, Eli Douglas, arrived in Galveston and began modernizing and reorganizing a fairly traditional school system with the aid of federal grants. Among the congregation of Douglas's church was Dr. Warren Dodge, a pediatrician at one of the Medical Branch's clinics. Douglas began to discuss with Dodge the possibility of the Medical Branch becoming health consultant for the school system. "If we want our children to become better educated," theorized Douglas, "we need to improve their health."

Mildred Williamson recently had joined GISD as coordinator of health services. A former Army nurse, she previously worked in public health in the Houston ghettos and also served as a school health consultant. Williamson had considerable experience in bringing health care to the people as opposed to bringing the people to health care. She says, "All the innovative components we eventually brought to Galveston including nurse practitioners, health aides, home school agents, and a shared record system had been in use in Houston beginning in 1971 when we received a federal grant from the Department of Health, Education, and Welfare." She served as director of that project in Houston for three years.

Dodge and Williamson began to apply for federal and private grants to obtain funding for the school health system they hoped to initiate. At the same time they began meeting with people in the community, asking questions such as: What do you really expect from a health service? Do you want only Band-Aids, or do you expect something more?

In the meantime, on a grant-seeking trip to Washington, Douglas and Dodge became acquainted with Philip Nader, who was working in a neighborhood health center in Rochester, New York. He also was making trips to the nation's capital trying to obtain grants for his program. In addition, he worked with HEW, writing guidelines for their health nutrition project grants. When Nader tried to establish such projects in the Rochester school system he faced many roadblocks, so agreed to come to Galveston in 1973 as associate professor at the University of Texas Medical Branch and medical director for the Galveston Independent School District.

While fulfilling his military obligation with the U.S. Public Health Service, Nader learned of the need many Americans had for not merely medical care, but for good total health care. "It was something I hadn't learned in medical school," he admits. "There's a big community out there. I went around the country helping communities with measles epidemics. I saw poverty with my own eyes and I also saw bureaucratic blocks to the delivery of health care. I gained the confidence to work with the people in a community." Nader took a year-long fellowship in behavioral pediatrics at the University of Rochester School of Medicine, where he had attended medical school. For the next six years he held a faculty post there and also worked one day a week as a school physician, pioneering a unique school health program in Rochester.

In one of the Medical Branch's recent publications, Nader wrote: "We're out to explore and evaluate different ways of delivering health services. School health activities need to be related to the specific needs of children and the community. We also need to explore ways of helping families and children take responsibility for meeting their own health care needs and not merely make them dependent on services. If successful, school health could then become effective preventive medicine."

He continued: "Barriers exist, however, that work against both school health and primary health care in fully achieving these new goals of health promotion. These barriers are deeply rooted in the institutions of education and medicine, but they are not insurmountable. They are unwillingness to change traditional ways, territoriality, protective professionalism among child development personnel, lack of trust and communication between 'school people' and 'health people,' fragmentation of services, and bureaucracy."

He added: "The physician should become part of the school institution itself in order to exert optimal influence. A closer relationship is indeed required. However, once he becomes part of the school system, he is then isolated from his medical, professional colleagues. If he were able to some degree to become independent, he would be able to operate more effectively. A useful relationship would be a marriage of the resources of school health and health care in a joint effort to accomplish their mutual goals—the health and education of children."

Early grants obtained by Douglas, Dodge, and Williamson permitted the development of a shared record system between GISD and the Medical Branch. A grant from the U.S. Office of Education led to the development of a health and nutrition project. It operated in five elementary schools with a high proportion of indigent parents. When that grant ran out after three years, Nader secured a grant in 1974 totalling $824,796 from the Robert Wood Johnson Foundation to continue some of the demonstration activities started under previous grants, but also to include a five-year plan to evaluate the impact of the newly emerging school health system.

There were two major means by which Galveston sought to upgrade its school health program:

1. Hiring health aides to work in the school clinic in conjunction with the school nurses. This freed time for the nurses and permitted them to obtain training to upgrade their skills and become nurse practitioners.

2. Hiring 10 home-agents to serve as outreach workers, who would function in the medical system as both child advocates and family advocates.

When Walter Dohl, president of our school board, visited Galveston with us, it was this part of the program that impressed him most. "They had people out on the street who could speak the language of the people," he commented, "yet still know what was happening in the school."

Of the 10 home-agents, eight had regular assignments in individual schools and two operated as "floaters," working where they were needed the most at different times. Williamson recruited the agents from local people who had backgrounds working in day-care centers, or had worked on the previously mentioned nutrition program, or had served on parent advisory councils. They tended to be individuals involved in community activities as volunteers. In their new jobs they often would be dealing with people from their own communities, families who lived next door, individuals with whom they had grown up, children who knew their children. Lois Jones, coordinator of the home-agents, told us, "I find that a family is more comfortable receiving information from a person in their community than from an outsider."

Several of the home-agents are bilingual, an important attribute because of the high percentage in Galveston of Mexican-American families, many of whom are either unable to speak English or to converse in it freely. "The home-agents have been particularly effective going to the hospital with families on their initial visit," says Jones, "and in interpreting what the doctors and nurses say to the patients. At John Seely Hospital, they have such a great flow of people coming through every day, there is very little time for the personnel to sit down and talk with a family in Spanish. If the home-agent is available, he or she provides this assistance." Among the nine hospitals on the Island, John Seely is the largest and also the one that deals more often with general, rather than specialized care. It is the hospital most frequently used by people utilizing the school health services.

Another important function of the home-agent is to follow up with parents concerning appointments made for their children at school. Sometimes a nurse will examine a child in school and refer him to a specialist at the Medical Branch. After making the referral the nurse can ask the home-agent to contact the parents to make sure they are aware of the problems, and maybe even invite them to come to school so they can participate in the evaluation of how to treat the child.

The home-agent also may know how best to approach a family. "With some families you don't go into their homes too often," admits Jones. "The home-agent, living in the community, may know that two governmental agencies have been bothering that family that week, so the agent may hold off because of the timing. A lot of poor people are so pushed around by various community action projects that they don't know which way to turn. Or they may be embarrassed because they are on welfare. I may know that this family is qualified for food stamps or Aid to Dependent Children (ADC), but they may be reluctant to admit it. You may have to make three or four home visits before they will open up, even though they need help badly. They are afraid you will let out their secrets." (Later, when we began to establish our school health project in Posen-Robbins, we would utilize the home-agent approach used so successfully in Galveston.)

School health services work with different community agencies in Galveston obtaining help for children and their families. Many families are unaware of services available and home-agents can help them through the bureaucratic maze that might have discouraged them from obtaining help. In addition, many private citizens regularly contribute money or goods to families in need; the home-agents know who these citizens are.

"There aren't too many social problems without health problems," says Delores King, the pediatric nurse practitioner at Rosenberg Elementary School. She adds, "We have children who come in here and complain of a stomachache. It's a true stomachache, but it's related to something else at home. It turns out to be a family situation. Maybe there is a divorce imminent, the family is bickering, and the child becomes sick because of it."

In one instance, a family moved into Galveston from another community because one of the children had had a heart transplant and the parents wanted to be near John Seely Hospital. The child had severe emotional problems after having gone through such extreme surgery, so the home-agent visited to see if she could help and to check on the medication. She discovered that the father was disabled, the mother could not work, their children slept on the floor, and the entire family appeared to be starving to death. The home-agent called a social worker for welfare assistance for the family and located private citizens who donated bedding. It was a delicate undertaking, because despite their poverty, the family had a great deal of pride. "We are not trying to take that away from them," said Jones.

On another occasion a child in kindergarten appeared at school at 8:00 a.m., but by 10:00 the teacher noticed him missing. The parents were working and unavailable at home. Early attempts to locate the child failed, so the principal asked the home-agent to aid in the search. The home-agent, upon arriving at the home, looked under the house and found the child hiding underneath. Eventually, she convinced the child that he had nothing to fear in school.

In still another family, the father was gone and the mother was in a hospital at the Medical Branch. Because of lack of money, the family could not afford to live in a hotel nearby, so they pitched a tent on the beach. When one of the children was missing one day, the principal asked the home-agent to check because the address given for the family was non-existent. She began asking her friends in the community how she might locate the family and finally found them in their tent on the beach, where a 16-year-old took care of four brothers and sisters. Eventually, the home-agent found them a place to stay. The mother has begun to recover, and the children now come regularly to school.

The nurse practitioners, health aides, and home-agents have close ties to the school district. Williamson explains, "All our nurses are paid by the board of education here. They are part of the faculty in each school. All the other personnel, which includes health aides and home-agents, are either paid in part by the board of education or by outside funding. But the outside funding is given to us as part of our total service. When you have this kind of an arrangement, you are part of the school family."

How successful has the Galveston program been in improving the health of children? Such improvements admittedly are difficult to measure, but one small study of the impact of school nurse practitioners (according to Nader) indicated that they sent home only half as many students because of illness compared to the previous school nurses. Most of the children in Galveston also have a higher percentage of immunizations than other communities in Texas. "Many children enter this area without immunizations," explains Jones. "We take them to clinics to get their immunizations updated, with the parents' consent, of course. Many times the parents are willing to have their children visit clinics because they are employed during the day and cannot take time away from work to get the child taken care of."

The immunization level in Galveston was 45% in 1971 before the start of school health services. In 1976 it had risen to 99%. Other statistical indicators show that the number of problems identified as requiring outside referral increased from 63 per nurse before the arrival of pediatric nurse practitioners to 132 the following year. The percentage reaching a source of care increased from 50% to 86%.

During our visit to Galveston, we were interested in looking beyond the statistics. In our meeting with King, we asked if she and the other members of the project were beginning to make a dent in the health problems of the community? She was cautious in responding, "I don't know if it's a very big dent, but I can say that the children I refer to physicians get attention. I believe it's because I'm able to assess them better than before I got the extra training." Later, she conceded, "I do think it's working."

In another conversation, with Guy Parcel, a health administrator, we asked if the children were healthier. He, too, was cautious, replying, "The closest you could come would be to determine whether or not children with identified problems are getting health care, as they are here. The assumption would be that if they get the health care, they would be healthier, but that's still a big assumption."

Jones admitted, "Follow-up is a big problem with us and with those at the Medical Branch. If people are very sick, they initially go and do something about it. When they feel better, they don't necessarily go back. So we have to make certain that their long-range medical needs are taken care of as well as their short-term ones. But follow-up is a problem not only with us, but with any place."

One of the home-agents we spoke with commented: "We feel it is important to stress the need here to work with the school and know how to communicate with the children, to know how to talk with their parents, and to plan together and to work together. It is no longer a matter of having the 'big doctor' come in and make a little diagnosis and everybody else does everything else."

Before leaving Galveston we had one final conversation with Nader. He summarized the advantages of the school health program in his city: "The thing we are trying at the project is to develop a program for school health based on what your conditions, needs, and resources are in the community. Some people would say certain schools don't need any health program. I don't think I would go that far. At the minimum, you need a very active program of health education and at least vision screening. There is no community that I can think of where the health system actually provides everything, especially behavioral and emotional problems."

In visiting school health projects in communities such as Cambridge, Hartford, and Galveston, we had uncovered good ideas and saw how those communities operated. The next big question would be, Could we take what we learned and apply it to our situation in Posen-Robbins?

Part IV: Making It Work

"It's Your Own Body"

As we examined the health programs of different school systems, and spoke with numerous health professionals throughout America, it soon became apparent that it would not be enough merely to provide health care, no matter how excellent, for the children of Posen-Robbins School District 143½. Medical treatment for children at an early age is one form of preventive medicine, but we wanted to take one step further. We wanted to teach children how to take care of their bodies before they became sick. Health education became a high priority item in our planning. We discovered, however, that health education in many sections of the country often is a low priority item.

William H. Carlyon, director of the Department of Health Education of the American Medical Association, was outspoken on this subject. He contends that many schools spend too little staff time on health education and rely too heavily on outsiders. He observes, "The promoters of the various disease agencies—the March of Dimes, the Lung Association, the Heart Association, to name only a few—need visibility so they approach the schools to put on programs. Since the people who head up these agencies usually are prestigious local citizens, the schools set aside assembly time and let them come in. The result is that the entire health education program consists of bits and pieces supplied by outside health agencies who are crusading for their own causes. Health agency personnel can be used as resource people, and some of the literature they put out is useful, but the schools should develop a comprehensive health education program from within and not rely on the 'disease-of-the-month' promoters."

Tacoma, Washington, has one of the most extensive school health education programs in the country. Of the 80 health personnel working under Dr. Roger Meyer, administrative director of the division of health for the public schools, half are full-time teachers who have been specially trained for health education. Nurses are used for health education in the lower grades, and trained health educators teach at the junior and senior high school levels. In addition, Meyer also teaches health education classes. "What we're concerned with is the fourth 'R,' responsibility," says Meyer. "Our health education program is designed to teach our students that they must be responsible for their own health."

But Donald E. Cook, MD, chairman of the school health committee of the American Academy of Pediatrics estimates that only about half the schools in the United States have health education. He states, "If we're going to cut health costs in this country, the best way is through preventive medicine, and school health programs can contribute greatly to this goal."

Recently we stopped by a sixth-grade classroom in our district in time to see a young girl named Cynthia roll a pair of dice. She came up with two sixes. "Yeah!" cheered her supporters, who were gathered around a giant diagram of the heart and major blood vessels outlined in red and blue tape on the classroom floor.

The lucky roll permitted Cynthia to move out of "home"—the left ventricle. Counting aloud, she stepped off twelve spaces, moving up, into, and through the arch of the aorta. Cynthia wanted her luck to continue, because she had a long way to go—down into the legs and back to the heart, then out to the lungs and back. Alas, her next throw was seven. "Oh, darn," she said. Her unlucky roll meant she had to take a "risk" card.

Cynthia picked a card from the file, and her expression fell. "For using cigarettes, move back five spaces," said the card. Joe, her closest competitor, rebuked her, "Get back there, Smokey!"

In most health education classes students will likely study the labyrinthine pathways of the blood. The heart and the circulation system are vital mechanisms, but few pupils comprehend them and fewer still enjoy studying about them.

But the children in Posen-Robbins—as well as in a growing number of other school districts—are more fortunate, thanks to the Elementary School Health Curriculum Project. The game being played by Cynthia and Joe is but one of many learning activities in that program.

The Elementary School Health Curriculum Project was started by Roy L. Davis, an official in the Bureau of Health Education, located in the Center for Disease Control in Atlanta, Georgia. But many groups of educators contributed to the project during its decade of development—most notably two Californians, Richard L. Foster, former superintendent of the Berkeley school system, and Helen Delafield. In fact, this approach to health education is often referred to as the "Berkeley Model."

In more ways than one, this is a *systems* approach to comprehensive health education. First, it is based on a systems design in terms of organization and procedures. Second, it systematically explores one major body system after another, beginning in kindergarten and progressing through grade seven. Here is the schedule of topics by grades:

Kindergarten, Happiness Is Being Healthy (the Teeth).
Grade 1, Super Me (the Senses).
Grade 2, Sights and Sounds (the Eye and the Ear).
Grade 3, The Body—Its Framework and Movement.
Grade 4, Energy, Nutrition, and the Digestive System.
Grade 5, The Lungs and the Respiratory System.
Grade 6, The Heart and the Circulatory System.
Grade 7, The Brain and the Nervous System.

Although the program focuses on one particular body system at each grade level, Davis emphasizes that the explorations take place in the broader context of first, the total individual (the physical, emotional, and psychological aspects) and second, the total environment (physical, cultural, and social). "We tackle real problems that affect real people, and we help students to arrive at decisions that will make a difference in their lives," explains Davis.

The program's major components are:
1. Teachers who have undergone a brief but intensive training course. They are confident that the method will work, because during training they assumed student roles to experience the activities for themselves.
2. A reservoir of resources, both human and material.
3. A climate charged with curiosity, discovery, and sharing.
4. Support from fellow educators (including administrators) and from the broader community.

Davis, who holds master's degrees in both education and public health, spent 10 years in public school administration and nine years in federal school health programs. Unfortunately—or fortunately—much of this experience consisted of getting acquainted with things that didn't work. Nineteen years of struggling to surmount lethargy, prejudices, and inadequate resources caused him to feel disillusioned. In fact, the typical reaction when you try to talk to many educators about teaching health habits to children is, "It sounds good, but it doesn't work."

Then one day Davis heard of plans for a new federal health effort that would include a program to discourage youngsters from smoking. For Davis, the program held a two-fold appeal: First, it would tackle a significant health problem. Second, there was the promise of two resources he previously had found either lacking or in short supply: funding and a positive conviction that health education can influence people in the way they think, feel, and act. Davis lost no time in joining the National Clearinghouse for Smoking and Health.

The Elementary School Health Curriculum Project made a modest start in 1969 in the San Ramon, California, school dis-

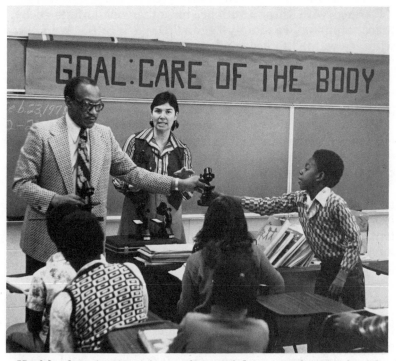

Health education is an integral part of the comprehensive health services in the Posen-Robbins schools. Teacher Isaac Baldwin offers student Eddie Mathews a microscope to view blood cells, a topic under study in a health class. Dee Clancy, health curriculum coordinator looks on.

91

trict. Although Davis was not sure at this time about specifically what he did want, he was well acquainted with some approaches that he wanted to avoid. These included:

1. Heavy reliance on the didactic method in presenting information or imparting values.
2. Overdependence upon textbooks.
3. Insistence upon covering all the bits and pieces of the conventional health curriculum.
4. Substituting compulsion for inner motivation in teachers or students.
5. Enlisting the teacher in a solitary effort, without the benefit of adequate resources or administrative support.
6. Concentrating on the child while virtually ignoring his cultural and social milieu.
7. Presuming that a person, if given sufficient facts, can be expected to adopt behavioral patterns that serve him best.
8. Looking to health education specialists to do the job. (For one thing, there weren't—and aren't—enough of them.)

"Armed with these cautions, but otherwise unfettered by preconceptions, we simply began," Davis recalls. "We knew what we wanted to accomplish, even though we weren't sure what methods would help us best achieve our goals. Our basic strategy was to develop models of success and use these to establish beachheads. The only way we could have national impact was through a rippling effect.

"We began in one district, relying more on by-guess-and-by-gosh experimentation than on formal, tightly designed research exercises. The things that worked, we held on to; those that didn't, we ditched.

"After three years, we enlisted a dozen additional school districts. Now, after nearly a decade, the program is being used in more than half the states. Actually, we aren't sure of the extent of its use, because we've trained so many teachers who have trained other teachers—and on and on. We don't mind this 'bootlegging,' as it were, as long as the basic elements of the time-tested mode are employed."

A school system can introduce the program beginning with whichever grade-level unit it chooses. In School District 143½, for example, we began with grades four through six, then added seven and eight. We soon plan to include kindergarten through third grade, thus covering all the years a child spends with us in elementary school. The training is offered to teams consisting of two classroom teachers, their principal, and one or two additional curriculum support personnel: nurses, health educators, curriculum supervisors, librarians, educational materials specialists, or others. Where there are enough trainees in an area to warrant it, instructors are brought in; otherwise, the trainees travel to designated centers. The team spends 60 hours in training, during which it works through the course, step-by-step and in sequence. In this way, the trainees experience the units as their pupils will. In our district the training occurred for two weeks during the summer, for three consecutive years involving three groups of teachers.

To be enrolled, the school system must commit itself to purchase about $3,000 in resource materials for each grade-level unit. (One set of materials can be shared by several classrooms during each eight-week to 10-week length of the unit.) The materials, listed in a catalog, are available from commercial, governmental, and voluntary association sources. They include a course guide, books, pamphlets, models, charts, filmstrips, films, tapes, and slides.

The same sequence of presentation is followed in each unit.

1. An introduction to pique curiosity, establish the importance of the study, and acquaint the pupils with the methods they will use.
2. An overview of the whole body and the relationship of its systems.
3. The structure and functions of the particular body system.
4. Diseases and other adverse conditions affecting the system.
5. What the individual and the community can do to prevent or control these health problems.
6. A culmination, or wrap-up, in which the students realign their thinking and share their newly acquired information and attitudes with each other, parents, and others.

The system encourages learning by doing—participation and sharing, individual and group initiative using a wide variety of techniques and media, and the involvement of many outside resources (visits by experts and field trips to interesting centers). An observer might, at various points in the several units, witness some of these activities.

For introducing the unit on the respiratory system, the teacher displays a "magic" black box and invites the students to guess its contents. There is nothing in it except air, of course. Now, having titillated their curiosity, the teacher encourages discussion of this ubiquitous substance; its composition and importance; how the human body utilizes it; the consequences of oxygen deprivation and air pollution; and whatever other ideas pop into the youngsters' heads.

The class divides into groups and visits designated learning stations. At the skeletal-muscular station, the youngsters cluster around a lifelike head and torso. "Hello," the plastic fellow greets them, "I am Hughie Humanoid. Can you take me apart? Can you find my lungs and take them out?" With enthusiasm and good humor the students proceed to take Hughie apart and then put him back together again.

At a blood bank, the pupils observe the operation of a centrifuge. A technologist displays the separated components. The whole cells, the youngsters have no trouble identifying—but this yellowish liquid stumps them. "It's plasma," the technologist announces. "Gosh," exclaims a plump lad, clutching the area of his heart, "I didn't know my blood had that sick-looking stuff in it!"

The classroom is transformed into a hospital emergency room, and the students pretend they are staff members and a variety of patients, one of whom is always the victim of a massive heart attack.

A visiting cardiologist brings cardiographic tracing and a take-apart model of the human heart. He distributes stethoscopes, including a school-owned instrument and others of his own, and coaches the boys and girls to listen to hearts and lungs in themselves and in their fellow students.

A veterinarian visits a class. Rather impatiently, the youngsters listen as he lectures on "How Animals Breathe." It's a good talk, but they are preoccupied with puppy sounds coming from a large cardboard box. The veterinarian produces the puppies; one is healthy, while the other has a congenital heart defect. The pupils listen to and compare the heart sounds. On his way to the school, the vet had stopped by a slaughterhouse. He brought along a mysterious mound of tissues, and somebody correctly guesses they're lungs. The vet invites the youngsters to look at, and feel, the spongy mass. He gets mixed reactions.

Firemen from a nearby station demonstrate resuscitation and other first-aid procedures. A pharmacist discusses common drugs, wonder drugs, and frequently abused drugs. He displays samples as he goes. A radiologist shows x rays of normal and diseased lungs. "If smoking does that to you, I'll never smoke another cigarette!" a boy exclaims.

The students consult dictionaries for root meanings of scientific terms, write thank-you notes to visitors, fill in crossword puzzles with words designating parts of the anatomy, design circular graphs to represent deaths from various causes, write essays on their individual health projects.

For Parents Night, students pose as a panel of experts and field questions from fathers and mothers, fellow class members, and teachers.

While each unit is designed to increase the student's health knowledge, equal emphasis is placed upon enhancing the student's sense of success and self-worth. Davis elaborates on this rationale:

"If you look at the major categories of undesirable student behavior—for example, cigarette smoking, drug abuse, problems with alcohol, and sexual misbehavior—a rather clear picture of the troubled and troublesome population emerges. Most often, the culprit is the kid who is considered a failure by the system and sees himself as a failure. This youngster is out of step and out of touch with his social environment. In his efforts to preserve some semblance of self-respect and to survive, he has tuned out all representatives of authority—the principal, the teachers, the coaches, the whole gamut.

"Now, if you want to encourage this boy or girl to adopt improved patterns of behavior—say, quit smoking—you certainly won't be effective if you employ a tactic that will increase his sense of being a misfit and will further estrange him from the system. You don't persuade a child to adopt better health practices by telling him what he must do, and especially not by preaching or scolding. 'Smoking is bad for you' isn't effective; does anyone argue that smoking is *good* for you? People simply don't act in a manner commensurate with their knowledge.

"In our program, we try to tune kids in. We present the youngster with a rich environment in which he can arrive at his own conclusions of what he wants to do and doesn't want to do with his body. We encourage freedom of expression, because we believe that, by and large, children decide for themselves what they will eat, and how much; if they will exercise, and how much; and whether or not they will drink or smoke, and how much. You cannot rely on manipulation; the boy or girl has to buy in—has to make decisions on the basis of his own authority.

"Also in connection with self-enhancement, we avoid use of artificial incentives. We would prefer to have a child experience wonder at hearing his own heartbeat than have him boast that he made an A in health. Our stance is, 'It's your own body, and it's important to you; it's your own value system, and it's worth giving serious thought to.' We stress peer education, and especially interpersonal exchanges when looking at adoption of life-style options."

The curriculum project also encourages interaction between the student and his family and community. Children are good agents for health improvement in their homes, and they're "culture changers" in their communities, Davis says. At the beginning of a unit, the student takes home an announcement about the course, its contents, the methods, and the desired results. Parent participation is invited. During the course, the student is encouraged to discuss health matters with his parents and siblings. If a youngster is studying about smoking, and one parent or both parents smoke, it may be unrealistic to expect the parents to quit, but it is realistic to expect them to engage in a dialogue with their child about this dangerous practice. In one family, at Christmas, the student asked his parents for a special gift: a pledge they would quit smoking.

It also is anticipated that children will take the information about good health practices into the community. Often, they will identify individual and public health problems and either suggest solutions or recommend referral agencies. In numerous emergencies, students who have been trained in resuscitation techniques have rendered first aid when the adults about them either didn't know how or lacked the courage to intercede.

From the community there are many citizens having valuable information, insights, or skills to share that can be brought into the classroom. The visitors vary in their specialties and affiliations, but most often they represent educational institutions, governmental agencies, professional societies, or voluntary health associations; for example, heart, lung, or cancer societies. Parent experts are especially effective.

Roy Davis notes that our advanced technology has presented us with both new assaults on our health and new opportunities for disease prevention, cure, and control. Some of the most critical issues of our day hinge upon how our health resources will be distributed. Particularly thorny are the questions of how heroic life-support measures will be allocated—to whom and under what circumstances.

"The 40-and-over generation isn't prepared to discuss, much less resolve, these vital and complicated issues," Davis says. "And few of our professionals—doctors, clergy, lawyers, government officials—are equipped for these debates. It is becoming increasingly important that young people be sensitized to, and informed about, principles of health—the methodology, the costs, and competing values. I'm also desirous that we capitalize on the current wave of interest in health maintenance and disease prevention."

The Elementary School Health Curriculum Project has spread rapidly because of the simplicity of its strategy and presentation. Any teacher is eligible for training. The team approach to training reinforces each participant's enthusiasm and commitment and ensures opportunities for the sharing of ideas concerning opportunities and problems.

During the year following training, the team is visited by one or more of their instructors; and after the year is completed, the teams are reunited in a review session. Each team decides how it will pass on instruction to another team in the system, hopefully in another school. Also, consideration is given to introducing another grade-level unit into the system, thus providing vertical expansion in addition to horizontal extension.

With a knowing smile, Davis notes that when someone walks into a superintendent's office with a request for a new program, the first response is, "How much will it cost?" He asserts that his program is a relatively low-budget operation, with a very modest start-up cost. "A couple of teachers get excited, and they get fellow educators and administrators excited, and you're on your way." Except for financial support of the team while in training, the expense is limited to the $3,000 for resource materials.

The effectiveness of the program is attested to by its spreading into hundreds of new school systems; by expressions of praise from educators, students, parents, and community leaders; and by the findings of several formal studies. Because students find it interesting, attendance improves significantly. One principal reported that the school nurse customarily spent many mornings rounding up truant children from nearby shopping centers, and the principal's office was busy with visits from problem students. While the health program was being offered, he said, attendance was at an all-time high and discipline problems were at an all-time low.

Teachers and students have characterized the health education activities as fresh, exciting, relevant, and rewarding. Some of the improvements noted include: increase in library use; broader, more enthusiastic participation in group activities; more sharing between the sexes; increased self-concept; more warmth and caring among the students; and an enhancement of social attitudes generally. In the formal studies that have been undertaken, the results have varied, but in several instances there was noted an increase in knowledge and understanding of health terms and principles and improvements in self-concept, social attitudes, and health habits, such as lowered incidence of smoking.

But from our point of view, Davis' health education program tied in with what we were trying to do in our school. The children first get information in their curriculum, but they also get good immediate health care. The nurse practitioners and physicians who treat them when they are ill can reinforce what the students have learned in school. Therefore, the two health clinics that we began to build in Posen-Robbins in 1977 and 1978 were, in one sense, two additional health education classrooms.

Posen-Robbins Today

"**D**id anybody hurt you, Dacia?" asked nurse practitioner Betty Hicks. The little girl with tears running down her cheeks shook her head. "Then why are you crying?" Dacia shrugged her shoulders as though to indicate she did not know why.

We had stopped by the new health unit at Childs School one morning in the fall of 1977 to see how things were progressing. Childs School is in Robbins. The unit there had been open for business since the previous March. We commented, "It looks as though you're having an active day." Hicks smiled at us, "You should have been here yesterday." A second nurse practitioner, Jim Williams, explained, "Yesterday was the day for the screamers."

Williams and Hicks provide primary health care for the children of School District 143½. Our dream, and the Robert Wood Johnson Foundation's dream, of a fully functioning school health program has become a reality.

The clinic and center of our school health program is located in a corner suite in the Childs School. Previously, the suite had been a kindergarten classroom, occupying 827 square feet of floor space. We redesigned and remodeled the classroom, which was no longer needed because of declining enrollments in the district. This medical unit accommodates our new health team, which includes, in addition to the two nurse practitioners, four health aides, a laboratory technician, and five health agents (our term for what others refer to as "outreach" workers).

The unit resembles a typical doctor's office. One enters into a small waiting room decorated with patterned wallpaper and paintings by a local artist. Beyond a glass partition is the secretarial area and desks where the health aides work. Off to one side are two treatment rooms. The unit also contains a wash-room and a small laboratory where our part-time technician spends four hours daily doing basic diagnostic tests. There are several storage areas as well—all this in a room that once housed a kindergarten class.

The cost of remodeling the classroom into a medical unit was $53,000. While we visited the unit that fall day in 1977, workmen several miles away were busy remodeling a similar classroom at the Posen School. It was to become the district's second medical unit. Because we had learned some cost-cutting procedures by the time we started the second unit and the architectural fees for duplicating what we had done once were less, the cost for this unit would be $37,000.

The layout in the Posen School was similar, but not identical to that in the Childs School. One change we made was to provide a wall, instead of a glass partition, between the waiting room and the secretarial area in order to provide more privacy for the staff when discussing medical matters. In one instance at the Childs School a mother had overheard two staff members talking about what she thought was her child's case and became disturbed because she felt she had not been told everything. As it happened, they were discussing another child, but the improved design in the second unit hopefully will avoid such misunderstandings.

One of the purposes for delivery of health care in the school setting, particularly with nurse practitioners delivering primary care, is to bridge the gap between patient and doctor. As mentioned in an earlier chapter, there are patients with problems and doctors with medical knowledge, but they are not necessarily getting together. Hicks explains, "There's a law in Illinois that says your child must have a physical examination before being admitted to school and again in the fifth grade. So because it was a legal requirement, the children of the district had gone to physicians for their examinations. Their problems were identified, but the parents didn't have a regular relationship with the physician, so they never went back. The physical examination record and the child were in the school, but the problem was never resolved. It's my contention that it does no good to find problems. Anybody can find problems. We must be able to solve them."

Those problems now are being solved—and further problems identified—at our medical unit, which is open between 8:00 a.m. and 4:00 p.m. every Monday through Friday, not only while school is in session, but 12 months of the year. Four of those days (Monday, Tuesday, Thursday, and Friday), nurse practitioners Hicks and Williams give routine physical examinations to those who need them, as required by Illinois law. On Wednesday they work on administrative matters and also see any children who may be ill. On Tuesday Dr. Charles Bono sees any patients who may need attention beyond what the two nurse practitioners give. On Friday Dr. Eugene Diamond (who also serves as medical director for the unit), makes a similar visit.

At 10:50 a.m. on the day we visited the unit, Diamond arrived and hung his coat on the rack. Before seeing any patients, however, he sat down in one of the treatment rooms with the two nurse practitioners. He handed them a copy of an article he had obtained at a recent pediatricians meeting showing a form that could be used for screening scoliosis, an abnormal lateral curvature of the spine. He also mentioned that he had arranged to provide an electrocardiograph (ECG) training session for clinic personnel at St. Francis Hospital in nearby Blue Island, the hospital with which Diamond and Bono are associated, and the first line of back-up medical treatment for the school health unit.

Williams had a quick question related to a 14-year-old boy

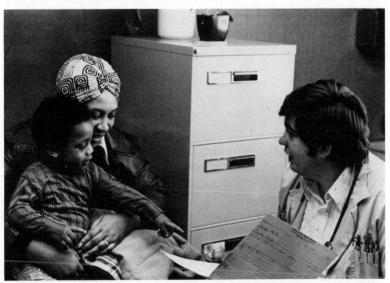

Communication with parents about the health needs of their children is a basic component of the Posen-Robbins School Health Project. School nurse practitioner Jim Williams has a consultation with Claudine Miller about her son Brian.

101

who was spilling excessive protein in his urine. Diamond answered it, then disappeared into the treatment room next door where a young patient and her mother awaited him. Meanwhile, one of the health aides was on the telephone trying to locate another patient who had an appointment to see Diamond, but who had not yet appeared.

Diamond saw his first patient shortly after 11:00 and by 11:40 he had seen four patients, averaging approximately 10 minutes with each, an appropriate use of his time.

With those visits completed, Diamond answered further questions from the nurse practitioners that they had saved for him related to patients they had seen on their own during the past few days. In a few instances, Diamond advised a course of action; in others, he suggested that an appointment be scheduled for his next visit. He also, in his position as medical director and chairman of the board of the corporation that supplies health care to the children of Posen-Robbins, dealt with several administrative problems, one concerning whether or not the laboratory technician, newly hired to replace a previous technician, was covered for malpractice under the corporation. Diamond discussed the question with the others, and decided finally that the technician was not covered. He suggested that she pursue the matter further through her association of laboratory technicians to make certain she was fully protected.

A year's malpractice protection for the laboratory technician costs $20. Nurse practitioners Hicks and Williams pay $25 annually for their malpractice insurance through the American Nurses' Association. Diamond, however, spends considerably more for his coverage since he is at least indirectly responsible for the actions of all the related medical personnel with whom he works.

Working with a nurse practitioner, however, may be a physician's best form of malpractice insurance. Many malpractice cases often are the result not of poor medical care, but rather poor communication. Patients resent what they perceive as brusque medical treatment; sitting long periods of time in a waiting room, then seeing the physician for only 10 minutes. They often are not involved in the discussions between different members of the health team before and after the 10 minutes spent with the doctor. One very important role of the school nurse practitioner is to provide a communications link between patient, parent, and doctor; to take time to explain, to educate, and to prevent future problems. "I spend more of my time with

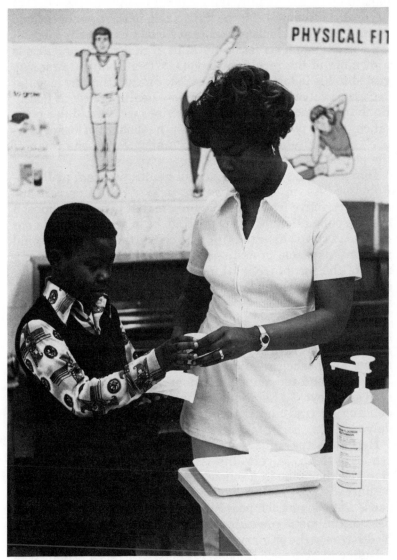

Health aides assist with many of the regular screening examinations. School health aide Valeria Bradley administers a dental mouth rinse to student Vinson Echols in Posen-Robbins' dental screening program.

preventive health than I do in the treatment of sick and injured children," says Williams.

The Posen-Robbins School Health Project provides care in stages. The first stage includes the school nurse practitioners working in the medical units near the classrooms. They are backed up by the pediatricians who are members of the staff of St. Francis Hospital. The pediatricians, in turn, are backed up by medical specialists available at Loyola University Medical School. Diamond serves on the staff at St. Francis and also is a member of the faculty at Loyola. When Diamond first suggested to his fellow physicians at St. Francis that the hospital become involved with the new school health project at Posen-Robbins, he met with what he describes as "formidable resistance." This "pseudo-indignation at the thought of loss of practice" eventually dissipated. "Fortunately I was chairman of the pediatrics department," he says with a smile.

Diamond talks about the school health program at Posen-Robbins: "As an efficient way to deliver health care, it has many attractive features. One thing is that you have almost a captive population. Kids are going to be in school every day or close to it, so you have the kind of access to them that you would not have as a solo practitioner, or even in a group. I'm cognizant of the sort of trivial things that might be overlooked, or disregarded, but could be of great significance if you know about them."

He discusses the relationship between nurse practitioner and physician: "I think all the subtleties of the relationship have not yet been worked out. There has been some tension in negotiations about such relationships. The American Academy of Pediatrics and the nurse practitioners' organization have not seen eye to eye. . . . Relationships will inevitably be resolved depending on trial and error and the personalities of those involved."

He favors the utilization of nurse practitioners within the school system: "It certainly is not possible to have pediatricians on the scene in a school system to deliver care. It would be unrealistic of me to suggest this as an alternate plan, because there is no such possibility. Given the need and willingness of the nurse practitioner to assume the responsibility of health care at the primary level, I would anticipate no problems."

Diamond also feels that St. Francis, which is a private hospital, has entered into the Posen-Robbins School Health Project with very altruistic motives. He feels that the hospital sees its participation not as a profit-making venture, but as a means

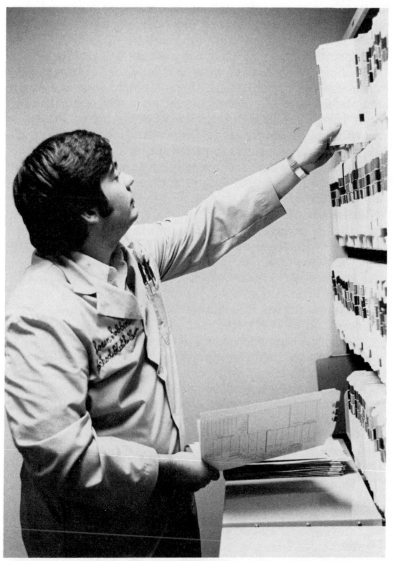

Comprehensive health care requires complete and cumulative health records. School nurse practitioner Jim Williams pulls a student's health folder in preparation for a consultation.

to fulfill a certain moral obligation to the general community it serves. If any financial advantage occurs, it may be in cutting down traffic in the emergency ward, which will ultimately save money for the hospital.

Getting the school health unit functional from the time it was decided to push forward with the project involved a lot of organization. In April, 1976, the Robert Wood Johnson Foundation sent more site visitors, including Beverlee Myers, formerly head of Medicaid for New York State, and Dr. Porter from Cambridge, to establish the need for a second grant.

One foundation request resulting from that visit was that Posen-Robbins obtain letters of commitment from the American Medical Association stating it would not oppose the project and from the Illinois Department of Public Aid stating it was willing to make payments to the school district. St. Francis Hospital contacted both organizations and within two weeks received letters of support. The speed with which we were able to obtain approval astounded us; most people seemed sincerely interested in our plans.

Rather than having the school district directly administer the delivery of medical care, a nonprofit corporation was established (with the aid of Kirkland and Ellis, a Chicago law firm). This was done for four reasons:

1. It prevented the school district from being the target for malpractice suits. Should a suit occur, only the nonprofit corporation would be liable.
2. It would be easier for a nonprofit corporation to be certified as a deliverer of health care than a school system. This would facilitate the project's approval by the mass of bureaucracies involved.
3. It would give the medical personnel involved a professional identity distinct from other employees of the school district. They could maintain their professional identity better in a separate corporation.
4. It would remove medical personnel from the regulations normally associated with school employees. Because of this contractual arrangement, nurses, for example, would not be subject, as teachers are, to tenure, unionization, and state teacher certification requirements.

At the end of the planning period, the Robert Wood Johnson Foundation decided not to include preschool treatment because it would be too great an investment at the start of the project. The foundation also suggested that the board supervising the health system be controlled by medical people. It also wanted

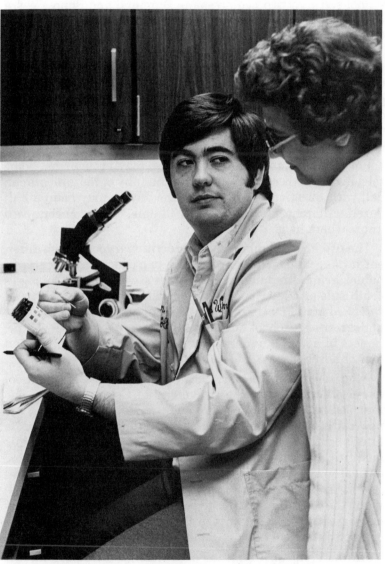

Posen-Robbins' medical lab provides many simple but important tests for medical diagnosis. School nurse practitioner Jim Williams discusses a urinalysis test with clinic aide Pat Calich.

the program to operate for 12 months a year instead of following the normal nine-month school year. These requests posed no great problems.

Perhaps the most important facet in the success of the health program at Posen-Robbins School District 143½ is the linkage between the two nurse practitioners, functioning within the school setting, with pediatricians Diamond and Bono. "We're in daily contact with them," explains Williams, "sometimes hour by hour."

Keeping in contact with the doctors takes skill, particularly with Diamond whose busy schedule takes him from one side of Chicago to another. Williams smiles when describing the ingenuity required to track down the two physicians, who, because they have office hours in the evening, sometimes take time off during the day. "You have to be a bit of a detective," he says. "You have to learn their patterns."

For Diamond that pattern includes staying near his home telephone between 9 and 10 a.m. so that any of his patients can call with questions. "The rest of the day he may be in a half dozen different places," says Williams, "but someone will know where he is."

The two Posen-Robbins nurse practitioners come from different backgrounds. Hicks obtained a bachelor of arts degree in public health nursing at St. Xavier's College on Chicago's south side and later received a master's degree in health and safety education from Indiana University. She worked most of her career as a school nurse in Gary, Indiana, with a few experiences in hospital nursing. Between her various jobs, she had four children.

After ten years in Gary, Hicks studied to become a school nurse practitioner at the University of Colorado. When she returned to Gary, she felt that she was not fully utilizing her new skills. "We were treating children under standing orders from about five doctor-preceptors, but we did not have clinic facilities. We worked in school nurses' offices and still were basically functioning as school nurses. The rest of the time we served as consultants for people with learning problems." When the opportunity came to become more involved in the primary treatment of patients in Posen-Robbins, she accepted a position in School District 143½, commuting daily from Gary.

Jim Williams also came to Posen-Robbins after working in a school district where he felt he was unable to utilize all his training. He graduated from Graceland College in Iowa, then went to work as a nurse in the Des Moines school system. He later took his nurse practitioner training at Rutgers University. In Des Moines, he had traveled from school to school on a rotating basis, giving physical examinations to all the children in the district. "We did nothing more than find problems, then tell the school nurse," he explains. "It was up to them to follow through and solve the problems. It was a very large district and it was impossible for us to visit each school more than once. We were merely scratching the surface. It was very unsatisfactory for me." He states about his new position in Posen-Robbins, "This system is designed so we can go that one step further."

He also adds that part of the problem in Des Moines was the relationship between the nurse practitioners, their physician-preceptors, and the other local pediatricians. "They [the physician-preceptors] were fearful of stepping on the toes of the other physicians. They were also fearful of malpractice."

In contrast, Posen-Robbins goes much further, invading, in one sense, the niche previously considered the private domain of licensed physicians. As one example, consider the laboratory where a few simple, but important, tests can be done on the spot and without delay by our resident laboratory technician Barbara Boetscher. According to Williams, "A lot of doctors' offices don't get involved in the type of laboratory tests that we do, and definitely a school nurse would not get involved in the types of laboratory screening available to us." This includes both throat and urine cultures, although not blood cultures. More complex tests are done by the laboratory at St. Francis Hospital, which provides laboratory back-up in the same way that Diamond and Bono provide medical back-up.

But perhaps more important than a well-equipped laboratory or office is the personal care that can be provided by nurse practitioners who can take time to relate to their patients. "Just listening to a parent talk about his child can be a very important part of treatment," indicates Hicks. "We talk to them and say, 'Look, it's okay for you to sit down and work with your child, and let the dishes go. This will help him in school later on.' Sometimes something simple like that can be very important, but the average doctor in his office doesn't have time to talk to the patients or their parents."

The average length of time spent by a patient visiting the unit is 30 minutes, and Williams explains, "That's not 30 minutes out there sitting in the waiting room, that's 30 minutes of clinic personnel time. If you compare that with the normal time studies of a pediatrician's office, that far surpasses their time allotment."

Hicks adds, "It is school nursing in its most ideal form. We can really become involved in follow-up. If we didn't, we would be just like another doctor's office." Follow-up in some instances consists of working with students who are overweight. Once a week, usually on Wednesdays, the nurse practitioners hold a weight counseling session. They talk to students about the need for diet and exercise to maintain good health.

Another vital factor in health care is patient compliance. A patient who has an earache is told to come back, and if that patient does not come back (perhaps because the earache seemingly has gone away), someone from the office will be on the telephone with parents or call the child out of class to find out why. When a child needs to be immunized, a health agent will keep track of that child until the immunization is done. Intrinsic to the success of the school health project at Posen-Robbins is good record keeping, organized so that patients who forget to comply do not slip through unnoticed.

During the school year the unit's five health agents work under loose supervision transporting people to and from clinic, school, or hospital in what might be described as a modified social worker role. "Our health agents are members of the community," explains Williams, "people who have lived here and who are well known by their neighbors. This allows them access to a lot of homes that a stranger might not get into as easily."

The one critical question that people often ask relates to dollars and cents: Does the primary medical care provided by nurse practitioners Hicks and Williams cost more than people otherwise would be spending on their health? Or, does it cost less?

In terms of the continuing cost of the program to the school district, most of the initial expenses were in start-up costs—paying the salaries of the staff involved in the planning of the pilot program and paying for the construction of the necessary facilities. The three-year grant from the Robert Wood Johnson Foundation covered 80% of these costs and the school district was responsible for the additional 20%.

As we complete this book at the start of 1979, the program has become operational, and with foundation funding soon to be terminated, the school board has discovered no unanticipated expenses. Most of the cost of the program is now paid for by three sources: 1) Medicaid, 2) third-party payments, and 3) private payments from patients.

As to an actual dollar figure, Jim Williams dodges the question when you present it to him. "I don't know," he says. "We don't approach health care from a cost point of view. It may cost the same, but we feel the follow-up and care we give is better."

The Future of School Health in America

In 1969 Dr. Charles U. Lowe, currently special assistant for child health affairs and director of the Office of Child Health Affairs in the Department of Health, Education, and Welfare, gave the principal address at the annual meeting of the American Academy of Pediatrics. He offered his vision of school health, which was much more expansive than the pediatricians assembled at the meeting seemed willing to consider. As Lowe recalls, "The talk was not well received. I was merely trying to perceive a better way of delivering health services to kids."

He felt that school systems could, and should, handle the delivery of primary health services since schools are one of the stablest institutions in the U.S., probably more stable than the family. Further, the scope of a school health program can be determined by local option, based on local needs. But what role should the government take in providing health care for all children? This returns us to the central question of this book: What is the future of school health in America?

An interesting summary of the problem and a partial answer to that question is presented in a study prepared by the Office of Child Health Affairs called: *A Proposal for New Federal Leadership in Child and Maternal Health Care in the United States,* published in 1977. It begins: "Health care for America's 70.5 million children ranges from superb to nonexistent. For those children living in families that have a source of health care available, and the knowledge and financial capability to obtain it, the private health care system delivers the best care that modern medical knowledge can provide. For those children living in families that lack financial resources, but have available a publicly supported clinic that provides comprehen-

112

sive health care, and who have parents who know when and how to obtain care for them, the public system delivers care that matches, or may even surpass, the private system in quality and comprehensiveness."

This study continues: "The problem is that many of America's children, numbering five to 10 million, have no access to primary health care at all. Many others use the health care system only sporadically, rather than being integrated into a system of continuous preventive and therapeutic care. Many mothers, numbering approximately 250,000 per year, give birth having received little or no prenatal care. It is primarily these unserved mothers and children who account for the facts that 15 other countries have lower infant mortality rates than the U.S.; that wide discrepancies exist between races and socioeconomic groups in indicators of health status; that children still die from diseases totally preventable by immunization and proper health care; and that many adults suffer, as a consequence, from a lack of appropriate health care. *If a change is to be made in measures of our national maternal and child health status, the focus must be on bringing unserved mothers and children into a system of comprehensive health care.*"

The above italics are ours, since we feel that statement is very important for what follows. "Such a change will not occur spontaneously," the study goes on. "It requires a national effort with federal leadership, and a commitment to the cause of improved health for mothers and children. A special focus on the health needs of mothers and children is justified on a number of scores; there is an inherent national interest in promoting the health and well-being of the nation's future adults. The known techniques of preventive medicine have maximum effectiveness when applied to mothers and children, and the nation's commitment to equal opportunity for all makes it unacceptable for anyone to face adulthood handicapped by a preventable condition resulting from inadequate health care in childhood.

"Government action to promote the health of mothers and children has not been lacking. A multitude of health programs, beginning with Title V of the Social Security Act in 1935, have been enacted to remedy perceived problems. Some of these programs have had a remarkable impact in certain areas, but for a variety of reasons the combined effect of these programs remains insufficient to meet the health needs of the nation's mothers and children, and the programs have even generated new problems of their own.

"Any attempt to bring unserved mothers and children into a system of comprehensive health care must recognize the barriers that presently exist that keep them out of the health care system, and must develop means to overcome these barriers. These barriers are related to availability, utilization, and organization of health care.

"Many mothers and children are left out of the primary health care system simply because there is no physician or other health care provider in an appropriate location. Therefore, *the first goal* of any intervention must be to make primary health care providers conveniently available for mothers and children to use.

"Having health care providers available does no good if there remain barriers to use of their services. Lack of a means to pay for their services, lack of knowledge of the existence of such providers, or how and why the service should be used, and lack of means to get to the provider of care prevent use of these services just as surely as if that care were not available. Therefore, *the second goal* of any intervention must be to promote appropriate utilization of primary care services by providing a means to pay for services for all who cannot afford them, educating mothers and children in appropriate use of such services, providing the support services necessary to assure that primary health care, when delivered, is effective, and, most important, establishing a link between provider and recipient of care.

"Disorganization and fragmentation of publicly supported services often contribute to public confusion, discouragement, and frustration when attempts are made to use these services. The family that must go to five different clinics at five different locations to obtain health care is not likely to go to the trouble of seeking preventive services. Therefore, *the third goal* of any federal intervention must be to coordinate management at the federal level, and to consolidate programs and simplify procedures at the point of delivery of services."

Of course, to many people the suggestion that the only solution must come in the guise of "federal intervention" is a discomforting thought. There is a basic conservative strain in America, though not always voiced at the polls, that equates bureaucracy with inefficiency. The fear is that the federal government spoils everything it gets into.

Dr. John Marshall, director of community health services for HEW, discussed this fear with us. We had asked him during one discussion whether we might wake up 20 years from now and find health programs fully established in all our schools. He replied, "If you had asked me five years ago if that would happen, I would have said, yes, because it looked as though the schools were branching out, increasingly teaching kids to be socially responsible and getting into new areas. But during the last few years, there has been a reaction to that, and increasingly schools are going back to basics. I'm not sure if it's because they believe this is best, or whether it's because the people have taken a look at their property taxes, which are the primary source of funding the school systems. They rationalize by saying, what you need now is a strict disciplinarian with 40 kids in a classroom, and never mind the fuzzy-minded liberal who's worried about their development and wants only 25 kids per class, with a reading specialist, a science specialist, and now a health specialist."

Among the others aware of this apparent shift away from what might be called federalism in the school system is Dr. Charles Lowe, who sometime after his speech to the American Academy of Pediatrics came to work at HEW and began to establish, at least in his own mind, a list of priorities in the area of health. "High on that list," states Lowe, "was school health, but not in a traditional mode." During his tenure at HEW, he has discovered that, rather than the federal government applying solutions, action has begun first on the local level. He says, "Communities on their own are beginning to address the issues, and solve them, and with a great deal of local color."

He adds: "There is a very definite movement toward school health underway at the local level, and HEW is seeking ways to support that movement.... Programs are doing their thing out there, and everyone is coming up with his own ideas. The leadership is coming up from the bottom." He states finally, "It is a healthy sign that the genesis is in the local system."

Lowe made these statements soon after visiting a number of the more outstanding experiments in the area of school health, including Porter's project in Cambridge, Massachusetts, and our own medical unit. While visiting Posen-Robbins, he particularly seemed impressed by the strong community commitment to the program as evidenced by the full support of our school board.

The common thread running through many of these school health programs is the presence of the Robert Wood Johnson Foundation which, with the exception of Cambridge, has provided seed money for all of the major programs discussed in detail in this book (Hartford, Galveston, and, of course, Posen-

Robbins). Committed to the development of a viable school health system in America, the Robert Wood Johnson Foundation in 1978 announced a $5 million school health services program with sites in four states. Christine Grant of the foundation explains, "The general aim of the program is to encourage states to introduce nurse practitioners in school settings to provide a broader range of comprehensive health, medical, and dental care to children."

But one major question, which Lowe raised during his visit to Posen-Robbins, was, Would the school health movement be better served by being funded by private or public sources? What, indeed, should the federal role be in establishing school health programs in America? We decided during our discussion that one of the most positive effects the federal government could have—stated most bluntly—would be simply to get off the back of the local communities, to modify Medicaid, and to modify some of the regulations that make obtaining funds difficult. For example, there are 106 child health-related programs in the federal government, each having separate regulations, guidelines, and bureaucracy. This causes considerable confusion in developing programs for mothers and children.

Another possibility would be to set into motion some sort of federal activity to start comprehensive school health programs in America, in a sense playing the role in all school districts that the Robert Wood Johnson Foundation now plays in a few. But it worried Lowe—and it worries us—that if the federal government assumes too much initiative, the vital effect of community interaction might be lost.

Particularly important in everybody's minds is the question, How do you pay for school health? This question is extremely important since it comes at a time when budget-conscious school boards have cut back on many previously important school programs in the areas of art, music, and even athletics in an attempt to save money. This was the basic conservative reaction that Marshall alluded to in his earlier remarks. The trend in educational financing lately has been that everything except basic education must go. With such a philosophy today, it becomes difficult to justify the establishment of what, in effect, is a new "department," somewhat separated from the mainstream of the educational program. Nevertheless, money to fund school health programs is available provided the people interested in establishing those programs learn how to secure it. And the amount of additional money needed may be less than some school boards might think. The estimated annual additional cost to the federal government and the states for providing primary health care to presently unserved mothers and children (according to recent documents from the Office of Child Health Affairs) is between $1.5 and $2 billion. That amount can undoubtedly be reduced by making the present system more efficient, as well as by emphasizing preventive primary care.

In financing any form of health care, there are three basic types of arrangements. The first type is when the party being treated pays out of his or her pocket. The second type is so-called third-party reimbursement, where the money comes from private insurance companies. The third type is government payments under such programs as Medicare, for people 65 and over; Medicaid, for poverty groups; and Early Periodic Screening and Diagnostic Testing (EPSDT), the children's version of Medicaid. Current estimates are that there are between 12 and 13 million children eligible for health care under this last program.

At the present time in Posen-Robbins, in addition to support from the Robert Wood Johnson Foundation (whose funding was particularly important for start-up costs), we receive both the first (private) and the last (government) type of payments. We receive little, if any, third-party payments, partly because most of our work occurs in the area of preventive medicine and insurance companies almost never pay for preventive care. At the end of three years, we expect that the above payments will take care of 80% of the cost of the school health program with the school board responsible for the remaining 20%, a relatively small sum and less than many school systems pay in salaries to school nurses who do not give such comprehensive care.

The important point is that many school systems are paying large sums of money for their health programs and getting very little in return. They fund a school nurse who is bored, underutilized, and sits in an office checking dental records or doing other tasks that have minimal effect on the health of the students. So in funding a more comprehensive school health program, school boards need not necessarily commit themselves to major additional financing; they simply must rearrange the funds they already are spending or those that would be available to them through public resources. The only place where major additional cost would be involved would be those school systems that have no health services at all.

Dr. Marshall also said, "The future of school health in America today probably is going to be inextricable from the processes that influence the total picture of where schools will be in America. That gets tied up with two issues. One has to do with what is the basis for financing schools. The second has to do with folks' perceptions of what the schools are doing by way of socializing their children and assuming some responsibilities for their children that they think ought to be their own—even if they don't necessarily meet them themselves."

There is another important point made by Dr. Lowe during his visit to Posen-Robbins. He said, "We are now at a point when there is access to school space. Things have changed. We've built up for the post-war baby boom, and now we are coming down the other way. As our fertility rate drops, we are faced with empty classrooms and empty schools. I visualize these being . . . delivery sites for health care."

At the same time he adds, "I would caution against using the school health program solely for poor children. It should not be; it should be a program for all children."

On the horizon, given the mood of the present administration, America seems to be bound toward some form of national health insurance. Many people both within and without the health field are wary of such a move. If such a national health insurance program is designed only as a payment system like Medicaid, it will still fail to resolve the fundamental inequities and problems of health services design and delivery. Important in any plan to change the health structure of America is the necessity to reorganize our system of delivering health care so that it can be provided to those who need it.

At the present time there still are barriers between the school child and proper health care. Among those listed by the Office of Child Health Affairs are:

—Lack of consumer knowledge about when and how to use primary health care.
—Lack of funds to pay for services that are perceived as noncritical.
—Bewilderment about how to negotiate a variety of eligibility requirements in government programs.
—Lack of coordination among publicly supported health and health-related programs.
—Lack of choice of service sources that tend to remove incentives to maintain high quality care.

Another problem to be faced is that, despite its ubiquitous presence in the lives of children, the school system does not function—as do most hospitals—on a 24-hour basis, seven days a week. Schools close on weekends, for vacations, and during the entire summer. "If you are going to have comprehensive care, what happens to children who get sick during these periods?" asks Gwen Bates, a consultant with the Office of Child Health Affairs. "It is easy to say that you have a back-up facility, or a hospital, but that back-up has to be something that is real, something that people will go to, something used and tested, and something with which you have an understood agreement."

Bates also feels that each state education department must become more involved with school health in concert with state departments of health. Many states say they offer comprehensive health programs, yet the programs range from minimal health care and health education to isolated activities in individual schools. State leadership is sorely lacking. We must still depend on individual schools to tailor programs to meet community needs. Perhaps the federal government can play some role by focusing on the issue and at least providing some standards for school health programs.

When we talked with Jane Fullarton at the Office of Child Health Affairs, she stated that she felt that what had happened in the past decade in school health shows what can be done when people committed to an idea start to make it work. But she had serious reservations about the immediate future, having watched the federal government in action for 15 years. She feels that you cannot mandate innovation, that for the bureaucracy to become involved in school health would be to "screw it up." She was, however, in favor of funding demonstration programs with communities doing their own planning. What Jane Fullarton would like to see is more innovative models written up (as in this book) so that we can learn from their good experiences as well as from their mistakes and disasters. "Where possible," she states, "some seed and planning money should be made available to help such programs get started, but there also should be some built-in evaluation, otherwise we won't learn as much."

In looking over our modest school health program in Posen-Robbins, we feel a sense of pride in being part of this movement. The experiment at Posen-Robbins could take on an importance far out of proportion to the size of our own small system. In thinking of this we can't help but recall a conversation we had with Dr. Henry J. Silver soon after he visited Posen-Robbins to observe our use of nurse practitioners in the delivery of health care. Silver, of course, is a scientist as well as an idea man. He described how you could warm water that would permit it to hold a supersaturated solution of salt in a beaker. Even after the water cools the salt remains in solution. But often all you need to do is drop one salt crystal into the beaker and suddenly, as though by magic, all the salt falls out of the solution to the bottom of the glass. That single crystal of salt was the catalyst causing that action. "Perhaps you," Silver said to us, "can be the catalyst that can cause something equally spectacular to happen in the field of school health."

About the Authors

Godfrey Cronin serves as superintendent of Posen-Robbins Elementary School District 143½.

William M. Young, president of William M. Young and Associates, was formerly dean of education at Chicago State University. He designed the Posen-Robbins Health Model and serves as its project coordinator.

The authors have requested that all royalties from this book be donated to the Posen-Robbins School Health Corporation.

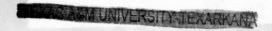